LIVING CHRONIC

LIVING CHRONIC

Agency and Expertise in the
Rhetoric of Diabetes

LORA ARDUSER

THE OHIO STATE UNIVERSITY PRESS
COLUMBUS

Library of Congress Cataloging-in-Publication Data
Names: Arduser, Lora, author.
Title: Living chronic : agency and expertise in the rhetoric of diabetes / Lora Arduser.
Description: Columbus : The Ohio State University Press, [2017] | Includes bibliographical references and index.
Identifiers: LCCN 2016040922 | ISBN 9780814213254 (cloth ; alk. paper) | ISBN 0814213251 (cloth ; alk. paper)
Subjects: LCSH: Diabetes. | Self-care, Health. | Medical writing. | Patient participation. | Communication in medicine.
Classification: LCC RC660 .A684 2017 | DDC 616.4/62—dc23
LC record available at https://lccn.loc.gov/2016040922

Cover design by Thao Thai
Text design by Juliet Williams
Type set in Adobe Minion Pro and Avenir
Cover image: WoodenheadWorld/Collection E+/Getty Images

9 8 7 6 5 4 3 2 1

CONTENTS

ILLUSTRATIONS

FIGURES

TABLES

ACKNOWLEDGMENTS

IN MANY ways this book began when my mom was diagnosed with what now is called latent autoimmune diabetes in adults (LADA). She was in her midthirties. My siblings and I were brought up with diabetes. We didn't talk about it. It wasn't explained to us as something that made my mom or my family different or not normal. We ate dinner at 6 p.m. every night and our iced tea was unsweetened, but otherwise we didn't really experience anything out of the ordinary. I thank my mom for that because this experience influenced the way I've thought about the disease and people with diabetes my entire life.

I have many other people to thank because, while books are often envisioned as being written in solitude, bringing such a project to light takes a village. I am lucky to have one such supportive village. Some of this support has been financial. For this I thank the University of Cincinnati's Taft Research Center, the University Research Council, and my own academic department. I also have colleagues who have given me the precious commodity of their time, offering to read my work and offer feedback. These people include Mary Beth Debs, Susan Allen, and Wayne Hall from the University of Cincinnati as well as my friend Heather Hall. But my village extends far and wide and also includes Jeff Bennett, J. Blake Scott, Lisa Keränen, and my fellow participants at multiple Rhetoric Society of America Summer Institutes as well as colleagues from the Rocky Mountain Writers Retreat—Kathryn Northcutt, Amy Koerber, and Kristin Bivens. I would also be remiss if I didn't thank Brian Still and the students in his 2008 usability class at Texas Tech University. Finally, I owe a debt to two anonymous reviewers who read my full manuscript and offered invaluable advice about ways to strengthen this final project.

I'd also like to thank Tara Cyphers at The Ohio State University Press for her unwavering belief in this project, the patient and thorough copyediting team at the press, and Daisy Allen Cunningham for her artful hand in capturing my vision of patient agency through her illustrations in the final chapter.

Perhaps most importantly I need to thank my study participants—the people with diabetes and health care providers who took time out of their busy lives to help me better understand how health care providers worked with people with diabetes and how people with the disease related to their disease, the technologies they use, their families and friends, their health care providers, and their diabetic community. I'd particularly like to thank Manny Hernandez, founder of TuDiabetes and the Diabetes Hands Foundation. Manny created a virtual space for people with diabetes to talk to each other, a space that was not attached to or monitored by a health organization. He also graciously welcomed researchers like myself into this space.

Finally, I'd like to thank my husband, Chris, for reading these chapters time and time again as they grew into a manuscript.

This book is dedicated to my mom—the funniest and kindest person I have ever known.

Searching for Agency in Chronic Care

"IT STARTS with an early morning blood sugar level," Tom said, describing what he does on a daily basis to manage his diabetes.[1] He continued:

> I am using a CGM [continuous glucose monitor], the Dexcom CGM. That does require calibration twice a day. I take that blood sugar level right away and then figure out what I'm going to eat for breakfast. It ends up being a struggle. I like cold cereal, but different cereals react better with me. . . . After I get to work, get settled, and have a break—two or three hours later—I do another blood sugar check then decide what to eat for lunch. That kind of thing continues. I haven't been doing as many pre-meal checks now that I've been on the CGM, but I'm still doing two or three hours after a meal and then correcting if I'm going low. I seem to bottom out later in the morning. I'm usually pretty active in the morning [at his job in a lab], doing a lot of running around, running tests working on products, so I usually have to have a snack to get me through some of that lull period. Then I follow that same trend, counting carbs, eating, doing a two- or three-hour-post sugar check.

Tom was diagnosed with type 1 diabetes three years before I met him. He participated in a focus group I conducted as part of my research in the lan-

---

1. Tom and the other names used for the people in this book are pseudonyms.

guage of patient agency in diabetes. When he was 27 years old, Tom's pancreas stopped producing insulin (the hormone that converts sugar, starches, and other food into energy), and now he injects synthetic insulin administered through an insulin pump.[2]

Although the management of type 1 can be more complex than that of type 2 due to the various technologies people with type 1 use (i.e., insulin pumps and CGMs), the tasks Tom describes are similar to those anyone with diabetes practices every day. The goal of all of these actions is to achieve near-normal blood sugar levels, which typically range between 70 and 110 mg/dL for a person without diabetes.[3]

Given the constant need for such self-monitoring, it is no surprise that patient agency, defined as the actions a patient takes outside of the clinical encounter to control blood sugar levels, has always been important in the discourse within the diabetes medical community.[4] This description of agency stresses notions of individual responsibility and autonomy that a person exercises after acquiring specialized expertise about the disease from medical professionals. According to medical and health care professionals, once a patient has received the necessary information, the person becomes an expert patient and possesses agency.[5] The term *expert patient,* a phrase often used for patients with diabetes, was coined by the United Kingdom's Department of Health following an observation made by doctors, nurses, and other health professionals that people with particular chronic diseases understand their disease better than a medical professional does. Even as experts, however, people with diabetes are encouraged to *follow doctors' orders* by doing things such as keeping scheduled appointments and taking medications as

2. Adults diagnosed with diabetes typically have been type 2, but there is a growing recognition that adults can be diagnosed with type 1 or latent autoimmune diabetes in adults (LADA), a more slowly progressing variation of type 1 diabetes.

3. The range of 70 to 110 mg/dL is typically used for daily blood glucose checks. The numbers associated with the diagnosis of diabetes are different and can be found in the American Diabetes Association's (ADA's) *Standards of Medical Care in Diabetes* (2016). People with diabetes may go as low as 30 mg/dL when they experience hypoglycemia and higher than even 400 mg/dL when they experience hyperglycemia. Both of these states can be extremely dangerous. In the short term, hypoglycemia can result in a loss of consciousness and a coma. Years of hyperglycemia can result in long-term micro- and macrovascular complications that include blindness, kidney failure, and cardiovascular disease.

4. Both the American Association of Diabetes Educators' national standards for diabetes education and the American Diabetes Association's standards of care use the term *self-management,* but the term *self-care* is often used as a synonym.

5. The Nursing Outcomes Classification (NOC) defines self-management as the actions a person takes to manage diabetes and prevent the disease's progression. The NOC is a standardized classification of patient outcomes developed to evaluate the impact of interventions provided by health care professionals.

prescribed. This troublesome relationship between compliance and expertise is, understandably, problematic for ideations of patient agency as an empowering concept in both the language and practices of diabetes work for patients and medical professionals. This tension is apparent in medical research literature in which, people with diabetes have traditionally been cast as a single, noncompliant patient set. As early as 1961, medical studies can be found characterizing study participants as "not well regulated" (Stone, 1961, p. 436). This trend continues into the current decade. A 1980 report in the journal *Diabetes Care* concluded that only 7 percent of diabetic patients adhere to all the steps of their therapy plans (Cerkoney & Hart, 1980), and a report five years later suggested that noncompliance rates for people with diabetes ranged from 20 to 50 percent (Harris & Linn, 1985). More recently, data from the third U.S. *National Health and Nutrition Examination Survey* from 1988–1994 and the *Behavioral Risk Factors Surveillance System* from 1995 found that 18 percent of participants from these surveys had A1C levels greater than 9.5 percent (Saaddine et al., 2002), and a 2011 study indicated that less than 50 percent of people with type 2 meet their target A1C levels of under 7 percent (Bailey & Kodack, 2011).[6] Health care providers, including those interviewed for this study, have echoed this belief that diabetic patients are, in general, a noncompliant patient set.[7]

This project started because of a nagging suspicion that such a singular view of people with diabetes does not tell the whole story. After all, as anyone with diabetes and any health care provider working with patients with diabetes knows, it is a complex disease. It comes in a variety of forms, including

---

6. The success or failure of maintaining control of one's blood sugar is measured by the A1C laboratory blood test. The A1C test (also called hemoglobin A1c, HbA1c, or glycohemoglobin test) gives information about a person's average levels of blood glucose (blood sugar), over the past three months. The test result is reported as a percentage; the higher the percentage, the higher a person's blood glucose levels have been. An A1C level for someone without diabetes is below 5.7 percent. Results for people with diabetes can be in the double digits; target levels are 6.5 percent (according to the American Association of Clinical Endocrinologists) or 7 percent (according to the ADA). And while the A1C is the gold standard of effectiveness measurement based on evidence from the *Diabetes Control and Complications Trial* (DCCT Group, 1993) and the *United Kingdom Prospective Diabetes Study* (UKPDS Group, 1998), more recent research (Skyler et al., 2009) suggests that this type of tight control may not be the best option for everyone and that A1C targets should be individualized. In 2009, an international expert committee recommended the A1C test as one of the tests available to help diagnose type 2 diabetes. Prior to that decision only the traditional blood glucose tests were used to diagnose diabetes (International Expert Committee, 2009).

7. Disability advocates and the new *Standards of Medical Care* from the ADA prefer the term *person with diabetes* to *diabetic*. I use the terms interchangeably simply in order to not repeat the same phrase too often.

type 1, LADA (also called type 1.5), type 2, and gestational diabetes.[8] It involves the complex endocrine system of the body, a series of glands that produce hormones affecting everything from a body's temperature to the ability to convert glucose into energy. Treatment involves working with primary care physicians, endocrinologists, dietitians, certified diabetes educators (CDEs), ophthalmologists, and podiatrists. Patients are advised to visit their doctors every four to six months for routine blood work and to see a foot doctor and eye doctor annually. With all these factors in play, it seems unlikely that a singular identity can characterize all people with diabetes—nor can the complicated work these people undertake to care for their bodies be represented as a simple process, as the biomedical definition of patient agency might suggest. A definition that is both rhetorically informed and interdisciplinary, as the one presented in this book, however, can capture such complexity. Such a definition does not work in opposition to evidence-based medicine but shares the ameliorative aim of other work in the rhetoric of health and medicine (see Scott, Segal, & Keränen, 2013).

THE EXIGENCE FOR A NEW DEFINITION OF PATIENT AGENCY

Long-term views of a singular subjectivity of people with diabetes create a situation in which it can be particularly difficult to *locate* the patient agency Mary Specker Stone began searching for in 1997. But the search for agency for people with diabetes, as well as other chronic illnesses, is particularly important now because of professional, social, and cultural shifts.[9] Foremost is the rising number of people living with chronic illnesses. According to the Centers for Disease Control and Prevention (CDC, 2016), as of 2012, about half of all adults (117 million people) had one or more chronic health conditions. By 2020, this number is projected to grow to an estimated 157 million, with 81 million having multiple conditions (*Lancet,* 2009). The numbers for diabetes alone are staggering: In 2012 a total of 29.1 million people in the United States (9.3 percent of the population) had diabetes (ADA, 2016a). The two main forms are type 1 and type 2. Type 1 diabetes affects approximately 5 percent of

---

8. Latent autoimmune diabetes in adults (LADA), or type 1.5, is an insulin-dependent type of diabetes typically diagnosed after the age of 35, often mistaken for type 2 at first.

9. In using the phrase *in search of agency,* I purposefully echo Mary Specker Stone's 1997 article "In Search of Patient Agency in the Rhetoric of Diabetes Care" in which she argues that in the United States, biomedical language used in texts developed in managed-care contexts constrains patient agency.

adults with diabetes (CDC, 2014). The other 90 to 95 percent of people with diabetes have type 2.[10] The difference between the two types is that in type 1 diabetes a person's body does not produce insulin, whereas in type 2 the body either does not produce enough of the hormone or the cells cannot properly use the insulin the body does produce.

Along with the exigence of the increasing number of people living with chronic illness are changes in medical practices and societal changes that privilege participating in discussions about health as well as taking actions to maintain health. In the United States, health care has been working through the kinks of shifting from a system that emphasizes compliance with doctors' orders to one that encourages patient-centered care and shared decision-making practices.[11] Unlike the traditional compliance model of care, the prevalent model for diabetes care since the 1970s and one that sets up a paternalistic relationship between doctors and patients, patient-centered care is designed to empower patients. In a shared decision-making model of health care, for example, physicians and patients are ideally working in a partnership that involves a two-way information exchange. At a minimum, the physician informs the patient of all information that is relevant to making the decision, including information about available treatment options, the benefits and risks of each, and potential effects on the patient's psychological and social well-being (Charles, Whelan, & Gafni, 1999). The patient provides information as well. This information includes her values, preferences, lifestyle, beliefs, and knowledge about her illness and its treatment. In these patient-centered exchanges, there is an expectation for patients to exercise a form of agency that is not only related to what they *do* to take care of themselves (i.e., taking actions that positively impact blood sugar levels) but also how they *talk* about their health.

Communicating about one's health (rather than passively listening to a doctor's advice) is also important in collaborative care, another emerging practice in contemporary health care delivery. In chronic care, these efforts

---

10. Although these are the official numbers of people with type 1 and type 2, people within the diabetic community argue that these statistics are inaccurate, particularly in light of the growing number of people with LADA. LADA accounts for roughly 10 percent of people with diabetes, making it likely to be more widespread than type 1 (Gebel, 2010).

11. As Segal (2009) pointed out, changes in language are not always matched by changes in practices. Although I have been unable to find statistics on the number of doctors that actually use shared decision-making practices, in conversations I have had with clinical researchers, doctors have noted barriers such as a lack of time and patients' statistical literacy levels to using shared decision making in practice. Therefore, it should not be assumed that shared decision making is a universal practice.

in part stem from the switch to the Chronic Model of Care in 1998.[12] This model was designed to overcome deficiencies seen in the practice of delivering chronic care, including the lack of time, care coordination, and follow-up (Improving Chronic Illness Care, 2016). The model includes collective entities such as the health system, the greater health community, community services, patients, and provider (or practice) teams rather than single practicing health care professionals. This collaborative approach and the increasing physician shortages in the United States have led more medical providers to experiment with shared appointments with one medical provider and several patients as a form of collaborative care.[13] These sessions might be for clinical care (checking blood pressure and doing blood work) or education about technology use (such as blood glucose meters and insulin pumps), diet, and exercise routines. In a University of California, San Francisco (UCSF) pilot study with group appointments, for example, a family physician and family nurse practitioner team guided six 90-minute appointments for patient groups that included as many as 15 people. The appointments included a 15-minute check-in, a *teaching period* with time for patient questions, and a one-on-one encounter with a health provider. During teaching periods, providers discussed a variety of topics, including nutrition, exercise, menopause, cancer screenings, and general self-care (McInaney, 2000).

The final factor creating the exigence for revisiting the concept of agency in diabetes is a societal change that places a high value on sharing knowledge as well as producing knowledge. According to a 2014 survey by the Pew Research Internet Project, people increasingly feel that the Internet and digital technologies improve their ability to share ideas as well as objects like videos or photos (Purcell & Rainie, 2014). People with chronic illnesses, specifically, are participating in online patient communities in greater numbers. When I began my own research with members of the online diabetes patient community TuDiabetes in 2009, the site had approximately 8,500 members. In 2015, the two social networks run by the Diabetes Hands Foundation, TuDiabetes. org (in English), and EsTuDiabetes.org (in Spanish), had over 50,000 registered members in total. In such online settings people talk about their personal experiences with the disease. For example, 66 percent of the Facebook

---

12. The model has been adopted by the board of the American Association of Diabetes Educators and the American Academy of Family Physicians. It is used in treating a variety of chronic conditions, including diabetes (Johnson et al., 2014; Atlantis, Fahey, & Foster, 2014; Howard-Thompson et al., 2013).

13. The U.S. Department of Health and Human Services projects that if the system for delivering primary care remains fundamentally the same as it is today, in 2020 there will be a shortage of 20,400 primary care physicians.

posts in one particular diabetic Facebook group described a user's personal experience with diabetes. Nearly 25 percent of posts shared sensitive aspects of diabetes management that were unlikely to come up in traditional doctor-patient interactions, including strategies for counting carbohydrates while drinking alcohol (Greene, Choudhry, Kilabuk, & Shrank, 2011).

Together, these four trends require a reconsideration of what qualifies as agency and expertise in the language and practices of diabetes. As Lynch (2011) reminds us, definitions are more than words creating meaning in a dictionary. They are, in fact, arguments (Perleman & Olbrechts, 1969) and "to choose a definition is to plead a cause" (Zarefsky, Miller-Tutzauer, & Tutzauer, 1984, p. 113). The cause pleaded for in this book is an alternative model of agency in the context of high-stakes discourses of diabetes. In such a model, people with diabetes are viewed as people doing work rather than people being cared for. This distinction enables agency to be visible in the first place. Once agency becomes visible, we see that it is a mutable, relational concept.[14]

This definition is informed by descriptions of agency in the fields of technical/professional communication and the rhetoric of health and medicine.[15] Although these fields are distinct in many ways, they also overlap and the lines between them are often porous. For example, scholars of health and medical rhetoric often find their academic homes in a variety of programs and departments, including technical and professional communication programs housed in English departments. Furthermore, their work is published in technical and professional communication journals.[16] Both disciplines also draw on rhetorical theory, and agency is a foundational, if contested, concept in both areas. This shared interest is particularly apparent in the vein of technical communication scholarship that draws on cultural studies and work in social justice.[17] In the rhetoric of health and medicine Segal (2005) specifically addresses agency within a compliance paradigm, characterizing this paradigm as inherently paternalistic and arguing that patients deserve "more respect than they

---

14. See Cooper (2011), Campbell (2005), and Grabill and Pigg (2012) for discussions of agency as emergent, protean, and fleeting.

15. Throughout this book, technical and professional communication is abbreviated as *technical communication*.

16. See the *Journal of Business and Technical Communication,* the *Journal of Technical Writing and Communication,* and *Technical Communication Quarterly,* in particular.

17. The list of scholars working in both technical communication/cultural studies and technical communication/social justice is too large to enumerate here. Examples of work in technical communication/cultural studies can be found in J. B. Scott, B. Longo, & K. V. Wills (Eds.), *Critical Power Tools: Technical Communication and Cultural Studies.* For examples of technical communication/social justice, see the work of Angela Haas, Natasha N. Jones, Godwin Y. Agboka, Lucia Dura, Michael J. Faris, Sara Beth Hopton, Kristen Moore, Dawn Opel, Gerald Savage, and Rebecca Walton, among others.

are typically afforded" (p. 141). Such stances not only offer the opportunity to critique in order to deepen our understanding of a situation but also open possibilities to intercede into what can be seen as problematic or ineffective practices. Such intercessions can be difficult to accomplish because they require shifting our gaze and questioning long-held assumptions. A rhetorically informed view of patient agency lends itself to such activities and is useful for resolving a problematic definition in the health work that people with diabetes and medical providers do, which can have a positive impact on health care practices and cultural understandings of diabetes.

OTHER LENSES FOR PATIENT AGENCY AND EXPERTISE

Broadly, agency has been defined as (1) possession, (2) authorship, (3) resistance, and (4) a relational concept.[18] The representation of agency as a possession goes back as far as classical rhetoric when Aristotle and Cicero centrally positioned the rhetor—a position that has continued through contemporary times, resulting in what Leff has called the "homage to the rhetor" (2003, p. 137). Western ideas about individuality have further spurred a notion of a *lone rhetor*. Together, these two aspects of agency—that of possession and that of the possession of a single agent—have created the problem of agency in the postmodern age.[19] Scholars in the rhetoric of health and medicine as well as technical communication have tried to broach this quandary by theorizing agency as authorship, resistance, or a relational concept. Technical communication's foundation in writing practices has encouraged a notion of agency as authorship.[20] Two particular areas of this scholarship have focused on the relationship between writing and agency: workplace studies and genre studies. Such studies examine the composing processes of engineering students (Selzer, 2004) as well as engineers in professional contexts (Winsor, 2003), the writing practices of former students transitioning into workplaces (Doheny-

18. Agency is divided into four discrete categories for the ease of discussion; these are not meant to suggest that the categories are mutually exclusive.

19. In her 2004 essay, Geisler summarized the conversations of more than forty scholars over four days at the fall 2003 meeting of the Alliance of Rhetoric Societies (ARS) about the question, "How ought we understand the concept of rhetorical agency?" Special journal issues in rhetorical scholarship that have focused on agency include a 2004 *Philosophy and Rhetoric* special issue and the 2005 forum in *Rhetoric Society Quarterly*. The Association for the Rhetoric of Science and Technology (ARST) also hosted a 2015 preconference honoring Carolyn Miller's work with the concept of agency.

20. The substantial scholarship on writing and agency in composition studies is beyond the scope of this book. See, for example, Cooper (2011) and Yancey (2011).

Farina, 2004), workplace professionals transitioning back into a writing classroom (Quick, 2012), and collaborative writing practices (Burnett, Cooper, & Welhausen, 2013).[21] Scholars interested in genre studies in technical writing also examine this relationship. Writing about the role of the genre of work orders, Winsor (2003) argues that the genre represents the relationship between the engineers (viewed as workers who create knowledge) and the technicians (workers who perform tasks based on the knowledge others create). Texts produced by the technicians, she argues, are not considered genre texts, or at least they are less generic than the work orders, largely because they are not visible anywhere but in the lab, even though many of these documents do order the technicians' work. Spinuzzi (2003) makes a similar argument in his book *Tracing Genres Through Organizations*. Here he states that most technical communicators view the user as a victim while the information designer is seen as a hero who is educated and provides better tools that free the user. Interest in these issues of power has continued to influence work in user agency as well.[22]

Writing as agency, with an emphasis on the act of writing and the relationship between author and text, can also be problematic in settings of health and medicine. Physicians and nurses and other medical professionals are authors of texts like prescriptions, educational pamphlets, research articles, care standards documents, and notes in patient medical records. People with diabetes who once recorded their blood sugar numbers, carbohydrate intake, and exercise by hand in diaries or logs no longer do even this type of writing. Rather, they take their blood glucose meter into a doctor appointment and the results are downloaded electronically.[23] Writing as a relational form of agency, however, does emerge within the spaces described in chapter 2. In these spaces, authors are not the source of discourse—authors, meaning, and knowledge are a function of discourse (Foucault, 1984b).

Scholars at the intersection of technical communication and the rhetoric of health and medicine have an interest in power and agency as well, oftentimes discussing agency as a form of resistance.[24] Koerber (2013), for example,

---

21. See Dorothy Winsor's work as well as Jim Henry's 2000 book, *Writing Workplace Cultures: An Archaeology of Professional Writing*, and Johndan Johnson-Eilola and Stuart A. Selber's edited collection *Solving Problems in Technical Communication* (2013).

22. See Hallenbeck (2012) and Rawlins and Wilson (2014) for other examples of such work in technical communication.

23. This process is not fully automated; people do have to enter diet and exercise information, but this is done electronically with the device.

24. Winsor also referred to agency as "resistance to authority" (2006, p. 441) and Herndl and Licona (2007) explored agency as a counterhegemonic action in which an agent can make her voice heard.

characterizes acts of resistance in relation to breast feeding messages and practices as disrupting the sense established by disciplinary rhetorics, a term Scott (2003) defines as "discursive bodies of persuasion that work with extra-rhetorical actors to shape subjects and to work on and through bodies" (p. 7). In rhetorical studies, the perception of agency as resistance arises in large part from Foucault's theory of resistance, which is related to his concept of power relations (Biesecker, 1992). In characterizing power relations, Foucault (1980) states that power relationships have two elements—the one with the power and the one whom power is being exercised upon. He outlines three elements of this relationship: (1) the primacy of a binary relationship between individual and other, (2) an emphasis upon the person who acts, and (3) the fact that a "field of responses, reactions, results" (Foucault, 1983, p. 220) creates the space for various actions.

In rhetorical studies in health and medicine, agency is a particularly thorny subject because of what Graham (2009) describes as "the often strict and authoritarian structures of Western biomedicine" (p. 378). And while resistance is an attractive definition of agency in terms of empowering people with little voice or power in highly authoritarian, expert structures, this way of theorizing agency is problematic for this study for two reasons. First, the study participants with diabetes did not voluntarily resist medical advice or assistance to improve their health, the most obvious form of resistance. In fact, they were engaged and informed and could see the benefit of good health. When I asked Tom about what he did to learn about the disease when he was diagnosed, for example, he responded in much the same way as the other participants:

> I started from scratch as far as doing carb counting, insulin levels, how to calculate basal levels, correction factors and all that. So yeah, I did that in a formal setting, but then that person also recommended three or four different books, so I went out and got all of those, as well as my own searching online. It was a combination of one-on-one educational meetings as well as my own reading and online research.

Along with learning from his health care providers, he took it upon himself to continue to find resources. Even Dan, the participant who seemed least involved in his care, still talked about going to the park to exercise when the weather got warmer and explained how a dietitian had told him that instant oatmeal can spike blood sugar levels more than Pop-Tarts.

> Pop-Tarts aren't as bad as some of the stuff that is high fat and long-term . . . Instant oatmeal does almost the same as Pop-Tarts. You wouldn't think,

but it's something about the processing and the chopping of it. I talked to the dietitian about it. If you eat real oatmeal, it won't do it, but who wants to cook real oatmeal over the stove?

Dan exercises options available to him. He does not resist advice nor does he blindly adhere to it, which might imply a "collapse of agency" (Armstrong & Murphy, 2012, p. 315). Rather, he processes the information the dietitian gives him and makes a decision about what he is going to eat, Pop-Tarts or oatmeal, by using both the specialized knowledge he has acquired and his own bodily knowledge of his food preferences and cooking habits, subjects taken up in chapter 3.

Agency as a whole in the settings examined in this project is a form of rhetorical work, which is attached to performances of expertise and enacted within a set of relations.[25] In using the term *set of relations,* I do not mean to imply a lack of connections as the term *assemblage* might. Nor does the term *set* imply stable connections—as the term *network* might by relying on a computer metaphor constrained by the ideas of information flow and linearity. Such a definition would mimic the one-way flow of information and linear sense of agency embedded in current biomedical definitions of patient agency. My model of agency contrasts sharply with a linear form of agency as defined in the practice of medical compliance, which provides a diminished model of agency because (1) it is based on the assumption that agency, like a possession, can be transferred from one individual to another (Martins, 2005), and (2) the term *patient compliance,* highlights physician agency rather than patient agency (Stone, 1997). Both concepts also emphasize autonomy so highly that a definition of agency as relational and shifting is impossible. Because of these limitations each chapter in this book draws on models from areas outside of medicine to explain the richer enactments of agency and expertise by people with diabetes.

A PRACTICE OF ARTICULATION

As I discuss in the following chapters, agency enacted by people with diabetes is a position occupied as a result of shifting identities and subjectivities within a network of material (bodies and space) and symbolic (discourse and

---

25. Both Herndl and Licona (2007) and Graham (2009) have argued that agency occurs with material-semiotic networks. Nodding to Latour (1987), Winsor (2006) also explored agency as an articulation of material-semiotic forces that includes "people, objects, facts, institutions, and whatever else can be made useful" (p. 419). Finally, Koerber (2006; 2013) argued that the acts of resistance function as a negotiation between various discursive alternatives.

texts) elements. To talk of agency with words such as *relations, performance,* and *space,* assumes that the speaker is an articulation rather than the origin of discourse. This notion is key to both how I study agency and how agency is enacted. To study agency I use a practice of articulation.[26] Articulation, as Stormer notes, is, along with other things, "about the formation of order, of the body and of speech, bringing together the material world, language, and spatial arrangement in one act" (2004, p. 263). Like Stormer, I see articulation as a performative practice. This practice, as argued by Slack,

> shifts perspective from the acquisition or application of an epistemology to the creative process of articulating, of thinking relations and connections as how we come to know and as creating what we know. Articulation is, then, not just a thing (not just a connection) but also a process of creating connections, much in the same way that hegemony is not domination but the process of creating and maintaining consensus or of co-ordinating interests. (2005, p. 114)

As a practice, articulation is useful for working with what Slack (2005) discusses as "arbitrary closures" (p. 114) and in situations in which linkages are not eternal (Hall, 1986). Articulation theory recognizes that these linkages are composed of material, social, and rhetorical elements arranged in material spaces. In this book, those spaces are those of online social networking sites and group educational/medical appointments. Within both these spaces, attachments are made, dissolved, and remade, giving us the opportunity to capture snapshots of agency.[27] Of course, all snapshots are not created equal and, therefore, are not all necessarily agential, as I also give evidence for in upcoming chapters.

MEANS OF AGENCY

To capture moments of agency and expertise requires acknowledging that agency is a "distributed, relational, dynamic, and temporal phenomena"

---

26. See Slack's (2005) use of the term *practice* in her historical account of articulation and its connections with cultural studies. Technical communication scholars and scholars in medical rhetoric have imported the term *articulation* from cultural studies (Grossberg, 1993) into their work to solve a number of problems. See, for example, Slack (2005); Slack, Miller, and Doak (1993); Scott (2003); Seigel (2014); and Koerber (2013). Additionally, in communication studies, see Greene (1998); Biesecker (1989); DeLuca (1999); and Lynch (2009).

27. In the use of the word *snapshot,* I acknowledge Scott's (2003) use of the same word to describe his way of studying the process of subject formation.

(Gries, 2012, p. 86) and recognizing that the physical experience of the disease is a constantly changing one.[28] To talk about agency in the contexts of a complex disease and a complex health care system, I rely on an articulation of interdisciplinary concepts. Together, these concepts—plasticity, liminality, and multiplicity—create the movement by which individuals affect change through adaptations in their orientations to other individuals, discourse, knowledge, and identities.

Rhetorical Plasticity

Agency is, in fact, a form of rhetorical plasticity made feasible in public liminal spaces (i.e., online patient community sites and face-to-face group appointments) in which multiple articulations of relationships are possible. Beer (1994) first used the term *rhetorical plasticity* in reference to reason in political discourse, but Gorsevski, Schuck, and Lin (2012) extend the term into scientific discourse in an argument that rhetorical plasticity explains how museum practices associated with the *Bodies: The Exhibition* museum displays evoked a rational, scientific discourse that ignored intercultural awareness and sensitivity. Other scholars have focused on more material aspects between bodies and plasticity.[29] People with diabetes do enact a form of bodily plasticity by constantly manipulating both their bodies and the technologies they use—insulin pumps and blood glucose meters (an idea elaborated upon in chapter 3).[30] They try to trick their bodies into working *normally* by injecting synthetic insulin or taking oral medications to replace the insulin their bodies no longer produce or use efficiently. They tweak dosages on pumps and program the codes associated with their test strips into their glucose meters. These material aspects of the disease have obvious material repercussions: They help evade short-term and long-term complications. But these actions also provide the capacity to become someone else: *Pumpers* become weekend sports warriors by decreasing their insulin dose and teenage girl pumpers skip insulin doses to lose weight and create skinnier selves. This bodily plasticity,

---

28. Gries (2012) undertakes this effort through the concept of rhetorical actancy, which she derives from Latour's (1999) notion of actant. She argues that rhetorical actancy acknowledges that "rhetoric is always produced from the dance of various actants engaged in intra-actions within various assemblages. The capacity to persuade, then, and to effect change is a distributed process created in the relationship between multiple and various *actants*" (p. 81).

29. See Jordan (2009) and Achter (2010).

30. Latour (1993) characterizes such human-machine relationships as *hybrids* and Haraway (1992) as *cyborgs*, a relationship between human, animal, and machine.

in other words, affords the ability to inhabit *multiple* subjectivities that are at once separate yet simultaneous.

Bodily plasticity is also intertwined with a form of plasticity that is at once rhetorical and social. It is rhetorical in that people with diabetes shift identities and subjectivities in relation to audiences and situations. This feature of rhetorical plasticity is similar to the notion of social plasticity in evolutionary biology, which refers to how animals monitor their environment and adjust their behavior according to their previous experience and the context in order to avoid negative outcomes, such as being ejected from their social groups (Oliveriai, 2009). Rhetorical plasticity also requires monitoring of the environment. Take the two Miss America contestants with diabetes as examples. In 1999 Nicole Johnson visibly displayed her insulin pump during the competition. In 2014, Sierra Sandison (Miss Idaho) did the same during the swimsuit portion of the pageant, later writing on her blog: "Miss America 1999 has an insulin pump, and it doesn't make her any less beautiful. In fact, in my mind, it enhances her beauty!" (Sandison, 2014, n.p.). Afterward dozens of people with diabetes posted pictures of themselves with their pumps to the Twitter hashtag #showmeyourpump. Both Sandison and the people following her on Twitter monitored their environment via digital technologies and adjusted their behavior in a manner that did not necessarily avoid negative outcomes but did create new opportunities.

Perennial Liminality

Most of the research in illness narrative scholarship, including that of Arthur Frank, describes the situation of illness as a threshold state between illness and wellness, one in which the person grapples with the disruption of an identity and refashions a new one—in the singular.[31] Such a characterization suggests a sense of permanence—a quality these identities do not share. They are, in fact, constructed and dismantled day in and day out through the process of testing. Testing in diabetes is a never-ending activity. It is done sometimes 4, sometimes 8 or 10 times daily. This activity reveals diabetes itself as a risky, liminal state, a term Lewiecki-Wilson and Cellio (2011) use to describe mothering in disability studies. For people with diabetes this risk is a physical one. They are at risk of losing consciousness, going into seizures, and dying from severely low blood sugar. High blood sugars can lead to ketoacidosis, which can cause diabetic coma or death. Less immediate but equally serious risks include heart

---

31. See Arthur Frank's extensive scholarship on illness narratives.

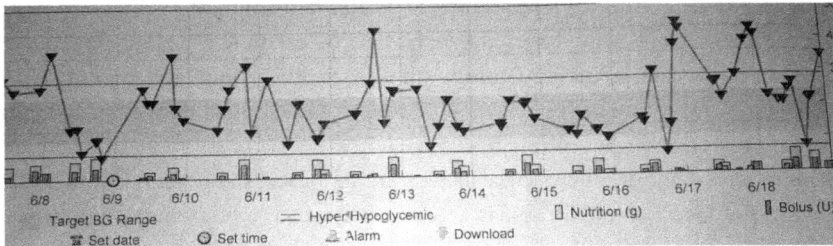

FIGURE 1. An example of blood sugar test results from a home testing meter.

disease and kidney failure if blood sugars remain at high levels for too long. People with diabetes also run the risk of being seen as *other*, a subject of anxiety and concern (Douglas, 1992; Lupton, 2013). Still, these mini-moments are not only tied to physical risks or actions such as eating a donut for breakfast or taking a walk for lunch—actions that do indeed impact blood sugar and change quite rapidly sometimes—but they are also tied to subjectivities and identities that people with diabetes inhabit, discard, and re-inhabit.

The chaotic pattern of the dots shown in the daily results of a person's blood glucose testing (figure 1) also illustrates that these risky bodies are "unpredictable" (Mol, 2008, p. 22). The nature of this unpredictability is one of perpetual or permanent liminality. Permanent liminality is an ambiguous state "neither here nor there, betwixt and between all fixed points of classification" (Turner, 1974, p. 232), but unlike the liminal state Van Gennep (1960) and Turner (1967; 1974) describe, permanent liminality does not cease once a particular threshold has been crossed, such as in the passage of coming-of-age rituals and marriages.[32] The type of liminality people with diabetes experience is similar to that which political anthropologist Agnes Horvath (2013) describes as the general condition of human existence in the contemporary world is "any situation where borderlines and boundaries that previously were stable and taken for granted are dissolved." (p. 10) and "events happen that are never ending" (p. 3).

Multiplicity

The nature of chronic disease as a state of suspended liminality makes multiple phenomena not only possible but, as Mol (2002) argued, enacted in

---

32. The word *liminal*, which is Latin for *threshold* or *doorway*, has been used in a variety of disciplines to indicate an in-between state of being (Bhabha, 1994; Lewiecki-Wilson & Cellio, 2011; Turner, 1967; Turner, 1974; Van Gennep, 1960).

practices that produce different realities. In her definition of multiplicity, Mol (2002) provides a complex characterization of medicine, saying Foucault's (1977) notion that medicine is unified has been abandoned and arguing that these days "we no longer believe in coherent sets of norms imposed in a single order" (p. 62). Mol's definition, based on her two years of studying the diagnosis and treatment of atherosclerosis in a Dutch university hospital, concludes that in practice a single disease is actually many and "a body may be multiple without shifting into pluralism" (p. 150). Multiplicity and the related concepts of liminality and rhetorical plasticity open up the possibility that agency manifests itself as a temporary performance as described in this book.

EARLY ATTEMPTS TO DIS-ARTICULATE AGENCY AND COMPLIANCE

Practicing articulation to understand agency in this particular chronic illness setting makes it possible to challenge deeply ingrained ways of thinking and ways of acting in the powerful discourses of health and medicine. Much as Haraway's (1992) essay "The Promises of Monsters" was a mapping exercise "through mind-scapes and landscapes of what may count as nature in certain local/global struggles," (p. 295), this book is a re-mapping exercise of agency through the articulations and dis-articulations of identities, subjectivities, material artifacts, and language in performances of agency. To begin this process requires loosening two *joints* that have become frozen in place. In other words, we need to *pull things apart* before *we put things together*. We need to pull agency apart from compliance, control, spoiled identities, and a narrative of progress for new articulations to become possible.

The compliance model has been a mainstay of the medical community's approach to diabetes from the time when insulin was discovered in the 1920s until the 1970s. Since this time, however, a number of efforts to redefine agency have been launched. One of these attempts involves replacing the term *compliance* with *adherence* in order to sever the implied connection to a paternalistic attitude toward the patient, to not cast blame on patients for not following physicians' guidelines (Chesney, Morin, & Sherr, 2000; Miller & Hays, 2000). It is important to point out, however, that while *adherence* is advanced as the preferred term, *adherence* and *compliance* are often used as synonyms. In their interviews and analysis of pharmaceutical and community-based texts, Mykhalovskiy, McCoy, and Bresalier (2004) found both terms used and often used interchangeably. My own interactions on multidisciplinary medical research teams confirm this assertion: In these informal conversations, the term *compliance* is still used when talking about patients.

In the early 1990s, another attempt was made to separate agency from compliance by a group of medical clinicians. These clinicians advocated for a conceptual framework of empowerment for diabetes patient education.[33] The framework follows Freire's (1993) definition of empowerment as being a way to freedom/autonomy. In other words, the focus is on increasing a person's capacity to make informed decisions rather than increasing a person's ability to follow instructions and comply with an authority (Anderson & Funnell, 2010). Other attempts to re-articulate agency have focused on language changes in terms of how patients are referred to. *Patient* comes from the Latin word *patiens* and means "I am suffering." As such, a patient is someone who is sick and cared for. In the late 1990s, doctors began questioning this term, suggesting that in an era of public involvement and active participation the word might be "an offensive anachronism" (Neuberger, 1999, p. 1756). One of the most prominent of these attempts to replace this anachronism in the United States has been the effort to refer to patients as *consumers*. A pharmaceutical video helps illustrate some of the problems with this particular characterization. In the YouTube video produced by the Animas Corporation (a company that manufactures and sells insulin pumps and related technologies), a narrator talks about the company's insulin pump. The narrator (a white male) begins by describing the cannula as "a fancy way of saying 'really tiny tube.'" The customer (a black female) remains silent throughout the short video as the narrator jumps past any technological discussion of this piece of computerized equipment to talk about the *skins* (cases) a patient can purchase for a pump: "And if I'm feeling flirty," he says, "I have a lot of colors to choose from." By skipping over the technological aspects of the pump, the video represents the patient/pump user as an uninformed consumer rather than a person who needs a high level of technical expertise to change the infusion sets, tweak insulin dosages, and calibrate the machine on a day-to-day basis.[34] The patient represented in the video is not concerned with the more technical aspects of the infusion set, such as the straight or angled insertion options the narrator

---

33. See the work of Martha M. Funnell and Robert M. Anderson in particular.

34. Most insulin pumps require the use of an infusion set to deliver insulin from the pump to the user. The set consists of thin plastic tubing, a cannula that is inserted just under the skin, and a plastic connector that joins the tubing and cannula together. The connector is generally mounted on an adhesive patch that is stuck to the skin at the insertion site to help keep the cannula in place (Rice & Sweeney, 2013).

describes in the opening. Instead, she is stereotyped as being interested in superficial characteristics such as color in making her purchasing decisions.

The problems that accompany consumerism as an ideology of excessive, unmindful consumption of goods was seemingly addressed through language with a change to the phrase *informed consumer* in health care discourse. Informed consumers make smart choices with their money. In health care, this characterization often translates into buying generic prescriptions when available or not insisting that the doctor perform a battery of expensive tests. In other words, the use of this phrase in health care is largely driven by a general effort to get people to be more aware of health care costs, making the assumption that this awareness will make people more careful about asking for or seeking these services. As both public and medical discourse would suggest, the term has become more pervasive since health care reform in 2010 in the United States. When the health care exchanges reopened in November 2015, for example, news articles regularly drew on language of the market and the concept of choice. In a *New York Times* article, the writer refers to people buying the plans as *customers* who shop (Sanger-Katz & Cox, 2014).

Informed choice is another term used to refer to both the exchange and understanding of information that helps a person make a knowledgeable decision. Within the framework of the Chronic Care Model used in diabetes care, the informed consumer is referred to as an "activated" patient. Interestingly, in the model the patient is still "informed" and "activated" by the medical community and the "prepared, proactive" practice team (Improving Chronic Illness Care, 2016). Viewing agency in terms of autonomy and freedom of choice assumes the inherent logic to the argument the health care community presents. The roots of this implied logic of science are deep: Weaver (2001) suggests that the belief in positivistic thinking in the nineteenth century induced "a belief that nothing was beyond the scope of its method" (p. 1352), a belief picked up by the medical and health care communities with little questioning. And while there are health care situations that require legitimate choice on the part of the patient, such as the choice of a birth plan (Owens, 2009) or in end-of-life decisions (Keränen, 2007), this view is problematic in terms of whether or not there is real choice in the rhetorical situation diabetes exists within. In diabetes care, the commonsense argument would go something like this: Eat right, exercise, and take your medications so that you keep your blood glucose levels stable; these actions will help you avoid complications like blindness and amputations, and you will lead a more productive and happy life. While we may accept these ideas as logical, choice is constrained.

RE-ARTICULATING *SELF-MANAGEMENT* TO *WORK*

As an alternative subjectivity of *patient* or *consumer,* I offer *worker.* The articulation of diabetes with work has implications for the relationship between
expertise and agency. As the opening comments from Tom suggest, people
with diabetes are not simply patients being taken care of. People with diabetes do a lot. Anderson et al. (1995) estimate that people with diabetes provide
approximately 95 percent of their own care in so-called self-managed tasks.
They test their blood, count carbohydrates, manipulate technological devices,
and monitor their exercise. All of this work adds up: In a study of 1,482 diabetic patients, Safford, Russell, Suh, Roman, and Pogach (2005) report that
patients in their sample group spent a mean of 58 minutes a day on self-care, or
approximately 363 hours a year. People with diabetes also often talk about the
disease as being "24/7" and "a full time job." These phrases consistently come
up in discussion forum posts in the patient online community TuDiabetes. As
a child, I watched my own mother, diagnosed with type 1 in her midthirties,
engage in this work. She would meticulously draw up insulin in a syringe twice
a day and inject herself in her stomach or hip. She kept hand-written records
of her blood sugar numbers, what she ate, and how much she exercised every
day. Later in life, when she and my stepfather would vacation in Myrtle Beach,
she did the same thing. There is no vacation from managing a chronic illness, rather, as Tom's opening comments and my recollections of my mother's
actions suggest, diabetes is constant work. In fact, Mol (2008) describes these
practical tasks that people with diabetes perform as "hard work" (p. 93).

And yet, the current discourses surrounding the practice of self-
management do not end up referring to the work a person does because it
gets enfolded into definitions of *care*. These definitions evoke images of a
sick person being administered to by the exemplary physician as healer. As
Malmsheimer (1988) states, "we have a cultural predisposition to hold the
entire medical profession in a kind of awe reserved only for those who fulfill
crucial roles in people's lives. Because doctors only are thought to be possessed
of the power to heal, to cure and to save lives, they only, among all professionals, are so thoroughly idealized" (p. 1). But diabetes can't be cured. It is managed or maintained. As such, while not necessarily oppressed by a dominant
structure, people with diabetes become marginalized in the practices and the
language of diabetes. A definition of agency that aligns with work ameliorates
this problem because such a model relates agency to value, a view the National
Institutes of Health have echoed in their reference to what caregivers do for
family members as "invisible work" (NIH, 2016).

If patient agency is a form of labor different from that of engaging in discrete tasks to manage blood sugar, what is the nature of this work? Mol (2008) suggests one definition in her discussion of care as something that includes technology rather than being in opposition to it:

> By unraveling the specificities of care in the case of daily life with diabetes, it is possible to disentangle 'care' from the all too immediate association with kindness, dedication and generosity. The point is not that kindness, dedication and generosity are irrelevant to daily life. They are crucial. But as long as care is primarily associated with 'tender love,' it may be cast as something opposed to technology. A pre-modern remainder in a modern world. Maybe such care can be added as a friendly extra, maybe it gets eaten up by technology, but in either case the two are mutually exclusive. But is this true, is care *other* to technology? (p. 5)

For Mol (2008), therefore, technology and care come together—and, I argue, they come together in what I call the work of diabetes. Mykhalovskiy et al. (2004) use the term *healthwork*—the purposeful day-to-day activities people undertake to look after their illness. In this study I invoke their term to replace phrases like *self-management*. Unlike Mykhalovskiy et al., however, I do not focus only on "people's purposeful day-to-day activities" (p. 323) as they take shape solely within institutional spaces such as doctors' offices and hospitals. My sense of healthwork draws in Conrad's (1985) notion of medication practice. Conrad (1985) looks at compliance in the case of epilepsy medication to argue that the patient's experience of illness and the meanings they attached to taking their medication is more salient for understanding why people are noncompliant than for looking at doctor-patient interactions to find these answers. In other words, both institutional work spaces and domestic spaces play a role in understanding healthwork. But because healthwork is changing, new and different spaces are now part of the landscape. These new spaces require additional definitional work as well. This work is aided by contemporary rhetoric and technical communication. Greene's (2004) work with rhetorical agency as communicative labor in particular is useful. Greene (2004) opens up the definition of work from a production-oriented view to one that includes what he characterizes as labor that is "often gendered and raced," but more importantly here, it is work associated with activities that take place "beyond the factory gates at home, in hospitals, in schools, and in stores" (p. 199). The work here extends Greene's definition of a workplace. Although Greene opens up this definition to include places other than the factory, the iconic space of production, his definition retains a binary explanation: Work spaces are factories or schools and work is gendered or not gendered.

Technical communication offers another appealing model that informs an understanding of the relationship between patient agency and work. This scholarship argues that technical communicators are symbolic-analytic agents, people who identify and solve problems and broker knowledge (Reich, 1991). Johnson-Eilola (1996) uses the role of symbolic analysts to relocate the value of technical communicators' work in the post-industrial age, arguing that

> symbolic-analytic workers rely on skills in abstraction, experimentation, collaboration, and system thinking to work with information across a variety of disciplines and markets. Importantly, symbolic-analytic work mediates between the functional necessities of usability and efficiency while not losing sight of the larger rhetorical and social contexts in which users work and live." (pp. 245–46)

Salvo, following Johnson's (1998) use of the term *technical rhetorician*, advocates for reformulating the technical communicator as a "professional rhetorical agent" (Salvo, 2006, p. 225). In medical contexts this might also be thought of in terms of critical awareness as Seigel (2014) and Emmons (2010) discuss. Similarly, Mol (2008) discusses people with diabetes as not just making choices about care decisions but making judgments, tinkering with technologies and relationships, and being adaptable and perseverant. Like symbolic-analytic workers and technical rhetoricians, the people with diabetes who were interviewed for this study use symbols and material to solve, identify, and broker problems by engaging in dialogues about their health. They simplify reality into abstract images that can be "rearranged, juggled, experimented with, communicated to other specialists, and then, eventually transformed back into reality. The manipulations are done with analytic tools, sharpened by experience" (Reich, 1991, p. 178).

In social spaces, the work they do as symbolic analysts requires that they negotiate materials (discursive and physical) not only to establish and maintain links but also to shift these links for articulations on an ongoing basis. These spaces help to move past binary constructions of the home or clinic and make visible articulations not only between the person with diabetes and her health care provider but between the person with diabetes and the disease, other people with diabetes, and diabetics' broader relationship to science and medicine.

TABLE 1. Providers Interviewed

PSEUDONYM	OCCUPATION
Daisy	CDE/RN
Kathy	Pharmacist
Amy	Pharmacist
Scott	Pharmacist
Susan	Dietician
Dr. Jackson	Primary Care Physician
Ken	Support Group Facilitator

LOOKING AHEAD

The story told in the following chapters about Tom, Grace, Sheri, and the other people I interviewed argues for a more fluid, multidimensional definition of patient agency than that of an act of successfully controlling blood sugar levels. Two particular collaborative spaces are investigated to make this argument: group medical educational visits and the patient online social networking site TuDiabetes. The texts analyzed include transcripts from interviews conducted with seven medical professionals and 14 people with diabetes (tables 1 and 2), 30 print documents used in group appointments conducted by the health care professionals interviewed, and 20 discussion forums in the TuDiabetes website. In recruiting and selecting people with diabetes for the study, the goal was to include people with type 1 and type 2 diabetes. Although the American Diabetes Association's *Standards of Medical Care in Diabetes*— the recognized guidelines for diagnosis and treatment of diabetes—recognizes four types of diabetes (type 1, type 2, gestational diabetes mellitus [GDM], and other types due to other causes, such as cystic fibrosis-related diabetes), historic and contemporary public discourse focus on types 1 and 2. I was also interested in capturing similarities and differences between interactions in face-to-face group spaces and online group space. Therefore, I recruited patients from a local physician's practice and an online patient community. When I began this project, I expected that the people participating in the online patient community would be much more empowered than the people who were basically *prescribed* the face-to-face group appointments. And yet, agency emerged in similar ways in these two spaces. Finally, in terms of medical providers, I wanted to show the range of the types of providers who interact with people with diabetes. The provider categories covered in this study, therefore, include physicians, certified diabetes educators, dietitians, pharmacists, and nurses.

TABLE 2. People with Diabetes Interviewed

DIAGNOSIS DATE	AGE	GENDER	TYPE	PSEUDONYM
1968	83	M	1	Norm
1968	50	F	1	Grace
1971	54	M	1	Dan
1974	53	M	1	Elliott
1976	57	F	1	Connie
1989	28	F	1	Sara
1995	26	M	1	David
2004	57	F	1.5	Terri
2005	60	F	1	Sheri
2008	30	M	1	Tom
2008	46	F	2	Mary
2008	47	M	1.5	Patrick
2009	33	F	2	Nikki
2010	42	F	2	Paige

Nine of the participants with diabetes were interviewed in focus groups (one session of four participants and one session with five participants). The others were interviewed. All but one of the provider interviews were conducted individually. In one case, two pharmacists participated in an interview because one was in the process of training the other. The focus groups were conducted and recorded online with members recruited from the TuDiabetes website. The individual patient interviews were conducted with patients involved in a face-to-face group educational/support group setting with a doctor, a certified diabetes educator (CDE), dietician, or pharmacist as the facilitator. The individual, face-to-face interviews were conducted in providers' workplaces and patients' workplaces and homes after the consenting process was completed.

To select my corpus of texts, I relied on the interview and focus group data to direct my selection of educational texts to analyze based on what the educators and patients said they used or recommended. More specifically, I used text from websites that both providers and patients identified as resources they had used or would recommend to someone else. I also used texts developed by the pharmacists for their company's disease self-management education (DSME) program and texts related to the Conversation Map program one provider used. The maps are part of the U.S. Diabetes Conversation Map program developed by Healthy Interactions in collaboration with the ADA and sponsored by Merck. They are used as part of an interactive game in group educational appointments in which a CDE acts as a facilitator. Patients use a themed game board to generate discussion and educate each other. The website texts (table 3) I included were from the following organizations:

- the American Diabetes Association (ADA),
- the Joslin Diabetes Center,
- Novo Nordisk's Cornerstones4Care educational program,
- The U.S. Department of Veteran Affairs,
- Merck's Journey for Control educational program, and
- the National Diabetes Education Program (NDEP).

My strategy for presenting an alternative model for patient agency involves using a dialogical approach (Emmons, 2010) to the texts I analyzed, putting the voices of diabetics and medical providers into conversation with each other in each chapter. This strategy is meant to honor voices by keeping them audible throughout the text, and these textual conversations act as embodiments of the juxtaposed and competing discourses of the liminal spaces I examine. In this case, these discourses are those of lived experience and clinical medical knowledge. Each chapter underscores and brings to light the vibrations between the materials in sets of relations in the processes of articulations and dis-articulations. Chapter 1 gives the reader historical background that articulates the narratives of care and technological progress used in the diabetes medical community to talk about agency and expertise. The chapter opens by establishing the importance of numbers in diabetes care in terms of their role in helping people with the disease to control blood sugar levels by testing their blood on home meters. After establishing the pervasiveness of the concept of control in the medical literature, extended examples from interviews with diabetics and health care professionals are analyzed to examine how the concept is taken up and used by people with diabetes. Chapter 2 examines collaborative spaces in which diabetes work occurs. The liminal nature of these spaces makes them ripe for enactments of agency and expertise. Such agency manifests itself through the emergence of counter narratives to dominant narratives of progress and control and through the act of writing as a social action.

Chapters 3 to 5 continue to explore manifestations of agency that occur through the mechanisms of rhetorical plasticity. Through an analysis of interviews and texts, the chapters look at patients' performances of agency in relation to subject matter knowledge, attributed expertise, and professional identities. Chapters 3 and 4 concern articulations associated with expert patient identities. Chapter 3 discusses the multiple types of knowledge production and knowledge sharing practices associated with expert patients. The

TABLE 3. Web and Print Texts Examined

TEXT SOURCE	TEXT DOCUMENT OR WEB PAGE NAME	PRINT OR WEB BASED?
AMERICAN DIABETES ASSOCIATION		
	Getting the News	Web
	Basics	Web
	Blood Glucose Control	Web
	Complications	Web
	Denial	Web
	Anger	Web
	Health Insurance	Web
	Statistics	Web
	Your Health Care Team	Web
	Medications	Web
JOSLIN DIABETES RESEARCH CENTER		
	Overview	Web
	Getting Started	Web
	Getting the Care You Need	Web
	Monitoring	Web
MERCK PHARMACEUTICAL/JOURNEY FOR CONTROL		
	Learning About Your Diabetes	Web
	Living With Diabetes	Web
	Healthy Eating	Web
	Active Living	Web
	Patient Tools	Web
NATIONAL DIABETES EDUCATION PROGRAM		
	Step 1: Learning About Diabetes	Web
	Step 2: Know Your Diabetes ABCs	Web
	Step 3: Manage Your Diabetes	Web
	Step 4: Get Routine Care to Avoid Problems	Web
NOVO NORDISK CORNERSTONES4CARE DIABETES PROGRAM		
	Diabetes Basics	Web
	Cornerstones of Care	Web
	Beyond the Basics	Web
	Diabetes Medicines	Web
	Care Plans	Web
U.S. DEPARTMENT OF VETERAN AFFAIRS		
	How Does It Help Diabetes Control?	Web
PHARMACY-DEVELOPED DSME MATERIALS		
	Target Your Numbers	Print
	Natural History of Type 2 Diabetes	Print
	Diabetes Basics Visit Summary	Print
	My Plan to Take Charge	Print
CDE CONVERSATION MAP MATERIALS		
	The Five Conversation Maps	Print

chapter begins with a discussion of the three types of content knowledge that medical professionals and patients use to encourage expertise (in the case of the providers) or develop expertise (in the case of diabetics) and moves on to examine specific website texts and interview transcripts to analyze how the provider texts and patient texts vary in the way people with diabetes negotiate different types of knowledge. Ultimately, the chapter shows that in liminal spaces people with diabetes shift back and forth between types of knowledge, an oscillation facilitated by a form of rhetorical plasticity.

Chapter 4 considers how patient expertise is established through attribution and interaction as well as content knowledge. The chapter draws on Burke's (1950) concept of identification and Collins's and Evans's work with interactional expertise (Collins, 2004; Collins & Evans, 2002, 2007) to explore the tension between views of people with diabetes as single, static subjects versus complex, multiple subjectivities. The chapter also gives further evidence for the journey motif by exploring multiple examples of the use of this narrative in materials on organizational websites, including the ADA's, and materials developed for patient education by both national organizations like the National Diabetes Education Program (NDEP) and local providers, such as pharmacists. These examples contrast to the way people inhabit more than one subject position and take on the roles of both patient and expert in different situations. As such, these roles become "points of temporary attachment to the subject positions" (Hall, 2000, p. 19), and this temporality operates as a form of rhetorical plasticity. By negotiating and renegotiating their positions within the discursive situation, patients challenge the assumptions about identity, power, and agency that are discussed in chapter 1. Chapter 5 completes the discussion of agential mechanisms through an analysis of mimesis, a form of rhetorical plasticity that acts agential through repetition. Whereas chapters 3 and 4 focus on the question of how agency and expertise are performed by expert *patients,* chapter 5 shows how relational agency provides people with diabetes access to professional identities that can move them *into* health care spaces as workers. To do so, this chapter draws on the divisional aspect of identification and mimesis as a strategy of rhetorical plasticity. The book concludes with a discussion of how the definition of agency constructed in this book can be useful in theorizing agency and for making changes to health care texts and practices in a way that mirrors the kind of agency people with diabetes perform. Such a model is particularly useful in new health care spaces that include group appointments, shared decision-making appointments, and other patient-centered spaces of health care in the twenty-first century.

CHAPTER 1

The Current Landscape of Agency and Expertise in Diabetes

It's not the numbers you dislike—
the 3s or 5s or 7s—but the way
the answers leave no room for you,
the way 4 plus 2 is always 6
never 9 or 10 or Florida,

—B. Snider, "The Certainty of Numbers"

IN DIABETES, patient agency has been grounded in a certainty of numbers, the concept of control, and the concept of a linear journey of progress. From a clinical perspective, control has been viewed as relatively unproblematic for people with diabetes (Naemiratch & Manderson, 2006).[1] Doctors and others advise patients with diabetes to change their diet, exercise regularly, lose weight (if they are overweight), and take prescribed medication to achieve blood sugar control.[2] This control is typically measured as a range that people work with their doctors to establish. The American Diabetes Association advocates for an A1C of 7 percent and a range of 80–130 mg/dL (milligrams per deciliter) before a meal. The target established by the American Association of Clinical Endocrinologists and the American College of Endocrinology is an A1C level less than or equal to 6.5 percent.[3] Evidence of control is estab-

---

1. I should note that by saying this clinical work is unproblematic I do not mean to suggest that physicians rely solely on guidelines. They are aware that diabetes is complicated. Therefore, they work with patients on an individual basis to try to attain the goals set for them.

2. Currently, people with type 1 diabetes are prescribed insulin, which they inject subcutaneously. People with type 2 diabetes might use insulin as well, but there are also oral medications as well as a class of drug called incretin mimetics, injectable drugs that improve blood sugar control by mimicking the action of the hormone glucagon-like peptide 1 (GLP-1). These medications include a number of options in several categories. See the glossary for more information.

3. To attain this A1C level, a fasting blood glucose would need to be less than 110 mg/dL and the two-hour postprandial plasma glucose (taken one to two hours after beginning a meal)

lished through the numeric results that doctors download from people's home glucose meters when they come in for appointments and the A1C test, which is typically performed in the doctor's office every three to four months.

Numbers, in other words, would seem to provide evidence on which to base logical decisions. But much like the middle and high school experiences Snider describes in "The Certainty of Numbers," living with diabetes is not an easy math problem. The speed at which a canoe floats down a river is dependent on variables such as wind resistance and whether or not the rower's arms are tired. A person's blood sugar levels depend on multiple variables as well. For example, did he stop to have lunch? Was he coming down with a cold? Did he just get divorced? All of these factors can influence blood sugar levels. If a person gets an A1C blood test and the value is 8 percent, the equation is not patient + 8 percent A1C = uncontrolled diabetic. It would look something more like this: patient + (flu episode over Christmas holiday + holiday eating patterns) – (exercise five days a week + 1,500-calorie diet plan) = numbers less than ideal. The fact that the disease is experienced differently by different individuals makes it unpredictable as well. As my focus group participant Sam said,

> We deal with it every day. And we're different every day. And we exercise differently every day. And we eat differently every day. You have got to take the responsibility of dealing with that, rather than have somebody tell you how to do it.

Diabetes, in other words, is predictably unpredictable (Leslie, 2008). While there are guidelines to follow for keeping blood sugar levels stable, most people experience peaks and valleys that are often unexplainable, as illustrated by a post from a member of an online community:

> I swear that keeping a toddler's numbers within range is like herding cats. We had a day yesterday where NOT ONE blood sugar test was within range. She doesn't seem to be getting sick. She ate what she normally eats and didn't really do anything different re: exercise. No stress that I could see. I guess some days are just like that. . . .

If the embodied experience of diabetes was not so unpredictable and agency was a simple matter of cause and effect or a simple math problem, loosening the knot between agency and compliance in order to re-articulate

---

would need to be less than 140 mg/dL.

it to other ways of knowing, being, and doing might be easier. But the connection between agency and compliance is, quite frankly, a tangled mess. Compliance is not simply a medical practice but a paradigm, and paradigms are difficult to shift. Kuhn (1962) illustrated this difficulty by describing a psychology experiment with playing cards.[4] In the experiment, participants are shown ordinary playing cards that are mixed up with anomalous cards, such as a black four of hearts. Generally, the participants saw what they expected to see (either the four of spades or the four of hearts) rather than what was there (the black four of hearts). Paradigms also are what we expect to see. They are so strong that we have trouble seeing things otherwise, and when an anomaly occurs a crisis begins that threatens the existing paradigm structure. Compliance is such a paradigm. In Trostle's (1988) words, in fact, it is an ideology:

> a system of shared beliefs that legitimize particular behavioral norms and values at the same time that they claim and appear to be based in empirical truths. Ideologies help to transform power (potential influence) into authority (legitimate control). Compliance is an ideology that transforms physicians' theories about the proper behavior of patients into a series of research strategies, research results, and potentially coercive interventions that appear appropriate, and that reinforce physicians' authority over health care. (p. 1300)

Paradigms and ideologies are accompanied by sets of terms that reflect them. When we select such terms we create a circumference, which acts as a rhetorical blinder (Hill, 2009). Burke (1945) refers to such words *god terms*. He argues that god terms work within particular epistemologies and their associated screens, a concept he uses to talk about the relationship between language and perception. These terms evoke a universal positive response because they are viewed through similar terministic screens that direct our "*attention*" (Burke, 1966, p. 45) by reflecting, selecting, and deflecting reality. To illustrate this concept, Burke (1966) provided an example from psychoanalysis, saying that if a person took a dream to a Freudian analyst, the interpretation of that dream would be different than an interpretation from a Jungian analyst or Adlerian analyst. The same dream is interpreted differently because of the education and philosophy of psychology that each of these analysts/schools adhere to.

---

4. Kuhn cites a 1949 study by J. S Bruner and Leo Postman, "On the Perception of Incongruity: A Paradigm," in the *Journal of Personality, 18,* 206–23.

In diabetes discourse, the terms *control* and *progress* have been organized and prioritized in ways that direct the language and behavior of both medical providers and people with diabetes. To dis-articulate these terms from agency, therefore, requires removing rhetorical blinders in order to make the original articulations visible. Then, terministic screens and the guiding principles and god terms associated with these screens can be re-articulated. This chapter undertakes this work of dis-articulating agency from compliance to begin shifting the terministic screen used to view patient agency.

CONTROL IN DIABETES DISCOURSE

The idea of control has always played a role in diabetes treatment. It is also a key term in discourses of diabetes. *Control* appears in medical journals on a regular basis (a search of the key words "diabetes AND control" in PubMed results in well over 100,000 hits) and comes up repeatedly in research outside of medicine, such as sociological studies of medicine.[5] The word *control* was not used regularly to describe a diabetic's disease status in the popular press until the 1950s, but it is such a powerful trope that it is capable of jumping from an established manageable disease (diabetes) to a new manageable disease (breast cancer): A February 19, 1956, *New York Times* article about a new drug to treat breast cancer, describes the drug as controlling (rather than curing) breast cancer "somewhat as insulin controls diabetes" (p. 65).

Control is also a constant in the conversations of health care providers and people with diabetes, including in the interviews conducted with health care providers and in the educational materials examined for this study. When asked to define *controlled,* one of the pharmacist participants related the concept to the referrals received from doctors, which are based on A1C numbers.[6]

KATHY: It [the program's referral criteria] used to say A1C above 8.5 [percent] for the referral. I think they took that off now so the doctor decides. They can check "yes, they are uncontrolled and they need this class."

---

5. See Broom and Whittaker, 2004; Heaton, Räisänen, and Salinas, 2016; Naemiratch and Manderson, 2006.

6. As used here, the term *referral* means the act of sending a person to another doctor or medical professional. Referrals are often needed in diabetes treatment for appointments with dieticians and certified diabetes educators in order for those appointments to be covered through insurance.

The National Diabetes Education Program (NDEP) and the CDC have used the word *control* in their educational materials as well. The CDC has a section called "Controlling Your Diabetes" in its book *Take Charge of Your Diabetes* (2003). The NDEP's diabetes education campaign—called Control Your Diabetes. For Life.[7]—used the word *control*[8] in its campaign publications that included "4 Steps to Control Your Diabetes," "Be Smart About Your Heart. Control the ABCs of Diabetes," and "The Power to Control Diabetes Is in Your Hands."[9] Even though such texts typically discuss healthwork as a team effort, which evokes a notion similar to a set of relations, it retains the nuances of autonomy because control language is so closely linked to the compliance framework of care. Furthermore, issues of power and physician authority remain attached to control in such discourse.

The idea of control permeates the language people with diabetes use as well. The Diabetes Stories oral history project, run by the Oxford Centre for Diabetes, Endocrinology and Metabolism (OCDEM), is an excellent example of this. The project includes over 100 interviews with people with diabetes, family members, and health care professionals. In an analysis of transcripts from 13 of these interviews, various themes related to control emerged, including blame, coping, and empowerment as well as control itself.[10] The theme of control was much more prominent than the theme of empowerment across the sample, appearing in 12 of the 13 interview transcripts. Even more interesting was the fact that of the 59 occurrences of a form of the word *control,* only 10 indicate the person in control of the disease rather than the disease in control, the doctor in control, or the disease controlled by outside mechanisms such as medicine or diet (Arduser, 2014).

The language of control was not absent from the interviews I conducted with people with diabetes either. Some of my diabetic participants related control to very specific and personal numbers rather than to general categories of controlled or uncontrolled diabetes. For instance, the following exchange

---

7. The punctuation used in the name of this campaign may be confusing, but it uses the period after the words *diabetes and life.*

8. It should be noted that these same publications on the NDEP's website used the term *manage* in place of *control* in 2016.

9. The NDEP is a federally funded program sponsored by the U.S. Department of Health and Human Services' National Institutes of Health and the Centers for Disease Control and Prevention. Established in 1997, it focuses on translating the science of diabetes prevention into clinical practice and on raising awareness among high-risk individuals, particularly those at risk of type 2 diabetes (NIDDK, 2015).

10. The 13 interviews I selected were from people diagnosed between 1980 and 2004, the period in which they would have had access to home testing meters and A1C testing.

came about when participants were asked how they had heard *good control* described.

> ELLIOTT: Well, for me, I'm a type 1 and I have been for 35 years, and I define good control as anything that is on a routine basis less than 100, and I define out of control [as] anything greater than 200. So, in that 100 to 200 spread, that's where the line changes for me. Somewhere in there, depending on the time of day.
>
> NIKKI: Well, I'm a type 2, and I control my diabetes with only diet and exercise. So I would say that for me good control is being anywhere from 70 to 140 milligrams per deciliters in my blood glucose numbers. I try to stay as close to normal blood sugar numbers for a person without diabetes as I possibly can without having any other detriment to my health or going low or just getting sick with any other problems, and that's kinda what I define as good control.
>
> PAIGE: I've been type 1 for 21-plus years. I would say good control is between a 6.5 and 7 A1C. I am thrilled and elated if I make it through a day with blood sugars between 80 and 150. I am rarely successful at that because of many other issues going on in life right now.
>
> SARA: I'm just on diet and exercise also, so I try to stay within a range of around 100 or less if I can achieve that fasting and no more than 130 to 140 at the absolute maximum at two hours after meals, and my A1C goal is less than 6 [percent].
>
> PATRICK: Yeah, I'm also a type 1 diabetic, late onset. I was diagnosed in 2008, so I'm still relatively new at this, but I define control for me as sticking in the 140 range. Generally I run 105 and I rarely go over 200, once or twice a month. An A1C below 6 [percent].
>
> ELLIOTT: I think mine is more reflective of the other type 1. I would expect on most days that I will be above 250 at some point, and at some point in the day I'll probably check in below 70, so my blood sugar is a roller coaster, and I take it that that's a little closer to what Sara does.

All but one of the focus group participants (Sara) began their answers by stating the type of diabetes they had. The three people with type 1 diabetes in the group—Elliott (the person in the group who had been diabetic longest), Paige, and Patrick (the newest diabetic)—moved on to describe how long they had been living with the disease.[11] After establishing this, they immediately began

---

11. Although Patrick self-identified as a type 1, the fact that his disease was late onset would classify him as latent autoimmune diabetes of adults (LADA), also known as type 1.5.

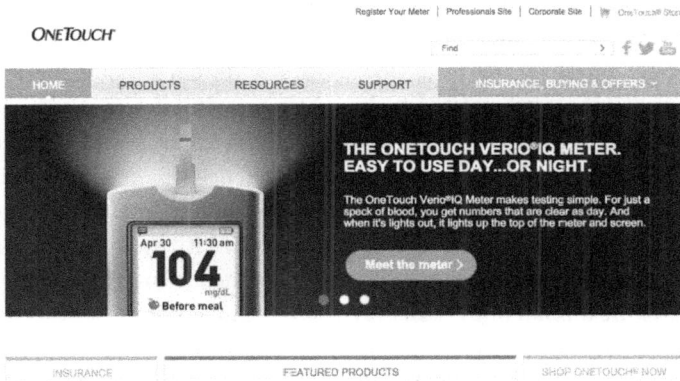

FIGURE 2. An advertisement of a meter showing a blood sugar reading.
Image from the LifeScan website.

correlating control to numbers, both the number they saw on their home glucose meters on a daily basis and the numbers from their A1C laboratory tests. The fact that these three participants did not mention diet and exercise does not mean that they do not use diet and exercise to help keep their numbers in the ranges they desire. It does, however, suggest that because a person with type 1 tests many more times a day (often eight to 20 times a day) than a person with type 2 (who typically might test up to four times a day), numbers are more constantly present in the day-to-day decision-making of a person with type 1. All the type 1 diabetics in this exchange started their comment by talking about blood glucose numbers. Nikki and Sara, who are type 2, however, started by talking about diet and exercise before talking about blood glucose numbers. Still, like the people with type 1, they ultimately define control through numbers.

SEEING THE NUMBERS

As these definitions of *control* suggest, the term is closely articulated with surveillance because the numbers that people are trained to control can only be managed through self-monitoring made possible through home blood glucose meters (and the A1C percentage). Watch any commercial about diabetes and you are likely to see the archetypal blood glucose meter (figure 2) showing a number in the good range, a blood glucose between 70–110 mg/dL. But *seeing* diabetes was not always a matter of making blood sugar visible as a number. The disease, which is widely referred to as an epidemic, was first recognized around 1500 BC by the ancient Egyptians, who considered it a rare condition in which a person urinated excessively and lost weight. In the second century AD, the Greek physician Aretaeus of Cappadocia declared that diabetes was a mysterious disease in which the "flesh and limbs melt into urine" (as cited in Feudtner, 2003, p. 4). It was diagnosed through an examination of this urine, a medical practice that goes back to medieval science when urine was almost the only diagnostic tool available to a profession that had "no firsthand experience with internal anatomy, no conception of electricity, germs or the circulation of the blood, and no instruments other than their own eyes to explore the mysteries of the human body" (Harvey, 1998, p. 1483). For most of its history, uroscopy was a visual science, but given the nature of diabetes, taste was also an evaluative tool (Feudtner, 2003). Early methods of diagnosis involved water tasters who drank the urine of those suspected of having diabetes because excessive blood sugar spills into a person's urine as well as blood. The urine of people with diabetes was thought to taste "wonderfully sweet as if it were imbued with honey or sugar," reported English physician Thomas Willis in 1674 (as cited in Rosenhek, 2005). This quality explains its clinical name *diabetes* (the Latin word for *honey*) *mellitus* (Greek for *siphon* or *flowing through*), but in the seventeenth century, diabetes was known as *the pissing evil*.

Eventually the diagnosis of diabetes moved from the sense of taste to that of sight, but urine was still the medium through which the diagnosis was made. According to Feudtner's (2003) history of the discovery of insulin, Matthew Dobson, a physician who practiced at the Liverpool Public Infirmary, made the first steps toward seeing diabetes in urine by using heat to evaporate the urine. Reporting on studies he conducted with a diabetic patient who had entered Liverpool's public hospital in 1772, Dobson stated that once he evaporated two quarts of the patient's urine, all that was left was a white cake that "smelled sweet like brown sugar" (as cited in Feudtner, 2003, p. 5). Blood sugar continued to be monitored through urinalysis, and as Clarke and Foster (2012) explained, throughout the 1900s improvements continued to be made to urine testing technology. In the 1960s, urine strips were developed for people to test their blood sugar levels at home. According to the American Diabetes Association, to test for ketones in the urine, a sign of high blood sugar, a person collects a sample of their urine, places the strip in the sample, and watches for the color of the strip to change. The tests are much like a modern version of the urine wheel that a physician in the Middle Ages would use to determine a person's health through the color of his urine. With the urine strips, a person compares the color of the strip to the color chart on the strip bottle. This gives a range of the amount of ketones in the urine. These were read according to color (e.g., blue meant there was no sugar present and orange meant there was). The color change was an effect of the sugar levels circulating in the bloodstream dumping into the kidneys.

In 1965 a team in the Ames Research Division of Miles Laboratories in Elkhart, Indiana, developed the first blood glucose test strip, the Dextrostix. The meter for the test strip cost approximately $495 and was only available for doctors' offices and hospital emergency departments (Clarke & Foster, 2012). As such, it was not until the mid-1970s that the idea of diabetics self-testing was contemplated. The Dextrometer, launched in 1980, was the first meter designed for home testing. The meter took much of the guesswork out of self-management at the time. Rather than getting a blood test once a week at the doctor's office, as my mother did in the 1970s, diabetics could—and were encouraged to—test their blood sugar several times a day. According to the 2016 edition of *Standards of Medical Care in Diabetes,* the charter document in diabetes treatment, most patients with type 1 diabetes or on intensive insulin regimens should consider testing before meals and snacks, occasionally after meals, at bedtime, before exercising when they suspect low blood sugar, after treating a low blood sugar, and before performing tasks such as driving. The guidelines go on to suggest that these actions would result in someone testing six to eight times daily, although individual needs may vary. The guidelines offer less specific guidance for people with type 2 diabetes because evidence is lacking for the connection between monitoring blood sugar and changes in A1C test results for this type of diabetes. In an exchange between members of one of my focus groups, this becomes clear as participants answer my question about how many times a day they test their blood sugar.

GRACE (TYPE 1): Oh gosh, 10 times a day.

PAIGE (TYPE 2): I test at least once a day, although my doctor said, "Oh, you could test twice a week and that would be plenty."

DAVID (TYPE 1): I test . . . my script is written for 10 times a day, but I usually run out before it's time for me to refill my script again. It usually happens—I like to do triathlons and I test A LOT whenever I'm training for those—when I'm on the bike, trainer, running, whatever, so um. I might use 10 just on a three-hour run, then I'll have another six or seven times that I test in a day. But then there's some days that it's a lighter schedule and I might only test four or five times through the whole day.

Once the technology of home meters and blood glucose test strips became available, people with diabetes not only learned to rely on numbers to determine their level of control as they performed the time-consuming tasks of self-managing their disease but they also learned to communicate about their disease through numbers. A personal example might help illustrate this.[12] While I was working on this book, a friend and I took our dogs for a walk. When I started the walk my blood sugar was 230, so I felt certain my numbers wouldn't go too low on a long, hilly hike through the woods. An hour later, feeling a little shaky, I tested and my blood sugar was 55. I explained my situation to my friend: "I tested before we left and I was 230, which is really high, but now I'm 55, which is too low. So I need to eat 15 grams of sugar [said as I shoved Life Savers gummies into my mouth] and wait 15 minutes until my blood sugar comes back up enough for us to keep walking." Not only did I rely on the numbers in terms of what I did in my self-management tasks, but I relied on them to communicate my situation to someone else. I had other alternatives that might have been more effective in talking with someone unfamiliar with the disease's "shorthand" of numbers—numbers standing in for explanations like "I might pass out if I don't eat something right now." And yet, I defaulted to explaining what was going on in my body with numbers.

Even people just at risk for diabetes use numbers to determine how much at risk they are. At a focus group about diabetes and storytelling with people in an urban Appalachian community, the certified diabetes educator (CDE) who was part of the research team brought brochures from the American Diabetes Association with a type 2 diabetes risk test. (The test is also on the organization's website.) The test leads a person through the following questions:

- How old are you?
- Are you male or female?
- If you are female, have you had gestational diabetes?
- Do you have a first-degree relative with diabetes?
- Have you ever been diagnosis with high blood pressure?
- Are you physically active?
- What is your weight?

Answers correspond to numbers that are then totaled. A total of five or more, according to the text, means that the person has an increased risk for type 2 diabetes. As our participants chatted before we began the focus group, they all filled out the test and compared their numbers with a surprising amount of interest, given that one of the things we found in earlier research was that people without diabetes who are at risk do not often perceive themselves to be at risk. This interest might indicate that tests like these will influence people who do acquire diabetes to communicate about their disease through numbers.

---

12. The author is LADA.

NUMBERS AND A SPOILED IDENTITY

Diabetics are not alone in this reliance on numbers, of course. Western culture in general has been heavily invested in the inevitability of numbers. In modern medicine, a certainty in numbers is related to a prioritization of science and evidence-based medicine (EBM), medicine based on evidence derived from the latest clinical research. This reliance is evident in medical literature as well as anecdotally. As medical practices moved from diagnosing diabetes through the general observation of sugar in urine to specific blood sugar numbers, practices in diabetes care also became grounded in this certainty. Providers use the A1C to determine what medications people should take or change, for example. They write prescriptions denoting the number of times patients test their blood sugar each day so that patients can get reimbursed for blood testing strips they use at home. Pay-for-performance health insurance plans use the A1C to determine how much to reimburse doctors for services tied to their diabetic patients.

The relationship between blood sugar testing and numbers also has consequences for how people with diabetes perceive themselves. In contrast to conditions such as high blood pressure, many chronic illnesses, like diabetes, are an *I am* disease rather than an *I have* disease (Pendry, 2003). *I am* illnesses include those in which attributions of blame for the condition rest with the individual (Pendry, 2003) and identity gets discussed in terms of the contradictory language of control, responsibility, and morality. An A1C over 7 percent can define a person as being a noncompliant, *bad patient.* People begin to internalize noncompliance as bad behavior, creating a spoiled identity in which they begin to morally judge themselves as bad. High blood sugar numbers reinforce this morality. Type 2 identities in particular are associated with morality, but the identities of people with type 1 are as well. Referring to type 1 diabetes, the Joslin Diabetes Center website makes the following statement:

> Leave behind the blame game. It is important for people with type 1 diabetes to know that they did not cause the onset of the disease, and that they are not to blame for being diagnosed with diabetes; this is especially true for children who have been diagnosed with type 1 diabetes. It is crucial that you periodically check in with your son or daughter to gauge where they are at in terms of understanding diabetes, and what they need to do to stay healthy. Remember that everyone deals with serious issues at a different pace, so if your child doesn't want to talk about how they feel right away, don't pressure him or her.[13]

13.

In public discourse, however, people with type 1 are more often cast in the role of victim. For much of the time since the second century AD, the disease was simply called diabetes. After a medical student in Berlin noticed some previously unidentified cells—later known as the islets of Langerhans—in 1869 and until after insulin was discovered in the early 1920s, diabetes discourse centered around type 1, or insulin-dependent diabetes. Prior to the discovery of insulin, diabetes was an acute disease that generally afflicted children and treatment was limited to dietary therapy that produced a semistarved state that typically ended in "coma, infection or starvation" (Feudtner, 2003, p. 6).[14] Narratives of the disease in the popular press, therefore, detailed the suffering of people with diabetes. A 1915 headline in *The New York Times* announced that Indiana Senator Benjamin F. Shively "suffers" from a septic form of diabetes (*The New York Times*, 1915, p. 13). Others with diabetes in the news prior to 1920 also suffered, had little hope of recovery, and often succumbed to the disease.

Interestingly, even with the discovery of a treatment (insulin), if not a cure, public discourse about type 1 subjectivities has remained remarkably stable. A 2012 *Washington Post* headline gives a current example: "Diabetes affects millions; society should not stigmatize its victims" (Sklaroff, 2012). Perhaps one of the most vivid contemporary images of diabetics as victims is in the movie *Steel Magnolias*. In the 1989 movie, Julia Roberts plays a young woman with type 1 diabetes who is about to get married. In one scene she sits in a beauty parlor chair getting her hair styled for the event and she experiences a low blood sugar. The scene shows Dolly Parton holding her shaking head so that Sally Field (Roberts's mother in the movie) can get Roberts to swallow some orange juice to counteract the low blood sugar. As Ferguson (2010) recounts, the scene is quite dramatic:

> Shelby is discussing her wedding arrangements at Truvy's (Dolly Parton) beauty parlor, where a group of friends often gathers. Suddenly, the soundtrack becomes echoic, the score shifts to ominously atonal organ, the camera moves to a close-up of Roberts's face, and viewers see Shelby become

14. Type 2 was recognized as early as 1875, but at the beginning of the twentieth century diabetes remained a single disease category and medical experts upheld the opinion that these patients had the same disease (Feudtner, 2003). By the 1950s, however, technical advances made it possible to measure the amount of insulin in a person's body, and clinicians were able to confirm that some patients with diabetes produced no insulin while others produced varying amounts of insulin (Rock, 2005). Attempts to standardize definitions, nomenclature, and diagnostic criteria around the world began around 1952 (Rock, 2005), and by 1979, the National Diabetes Data Group (NDDG) produced a consensus document standardizing the nomenclature and definitions for diabetes mellitus (NDDG, 1979). This document was endorsed one year later by the World Health Organization (WHO, 1980).

intensely out of control. She is panicked, rabidly tearing at her recently styled hair, fighting off her mother with fists as she tries to force orange juice down Shelby's throat before she finally recovers, sobbing in abject shame, "Oh momma I'm sorry," and apologizing tearfully to Truvy. (p. 184)

As depicted in this scene, Roberts does suffer. She is portrayed as a victim of her own body and as someone who needs help to bring her body back into control. In another movie, 2002's *Panic Room,* an adolescent Kristen Stewart acts out a similarly dramatic hypoglycemia-induced scene when she gets locked inside a panic room. In her case, she gets a Glucagon shot to bring her body back into control. These severe low blood sugars do occur, and people with diabetes may need to rely on another person to help them through such an episode. Less severe episodes are more common, however. Obviously the scenes in these two movies help create drama for movie-goers, but these portrayals also enforce a particular diabetic identity in our culture—a victim.

The public discourse surrounding type 2 is much more similar to the earlier quotation about blame and type 1 from the Joslin Diabetes Center website. Type 2, in contrast to type 1, is often characterized as an earned disease in both medical and public discourse. As such language focuses on issues of willpower and blame, as the following blog post illustrates:

Thing is, if I'm having a tough diabetes day, I blame myself. I'm the one who decides when to eat and what food to eat, and I'm the one who decides what exercise or other activities I'm partaking in for the day. I'm deciding when to test—and how often, and I'm the one who decides how much insulin to take, and when. I'm typing this as my numb tongue rests against the roof of my mouth. I feel vulnerable and shaky after my 2nd hit of low blood sugar today. A lovely 32 mg/dl and a previous 37 mg/dl. I rail against myself for not knowing better. Cleaning is exercise. Running two flights of stairs on and off throughout the night with heavy loads of laundry counts as exercise. Redecorating can't just be redecorating. It's an activity and basal rates must be adjusted. If not, you get *this.* What sucks most about diabetes from an emotional standpoint is all the guilt and blame that goes along with it. I can handle taking responsibility for things and I can even handle a healthy dose of guilt if it's "earned." Yes, I'll take the blame if it's deserved, but hell, I'm no pancreas, and a lot of these feelings of guilt and blame are not entirely mine to take ownership of.

Another example involves a recent conversation I had with a young woman who had gestational diabetes while carrying her twins. She described paralyzing feelings of anxiety as she watched the timer on her meter click down when she tested her blood sugar seven times each day. High numbers meant she was potentially harming her children. Obsessively, in order to be sure she was a being a good mother (by being a compliant patient), she would double check each time she tested to be sure the numbers were an accurate reflection of what was going on inside her body.

For people with type 2 diabetes high numbers also get translated as being fat and not taking care of oneself. One type 2 participant in my study made reference to this negative identity.

> MARY: When I was diagnosed and at 11.4 as an A1C, which, you know, in three months I brought it down to 6.5 and it's been below 6, but it's, you know, at that time when I heard that I thought, "Gosh, how did I let this happen?" That was my first reaction, and it's the psychological support that I really miss. Because the medical stuff, as you said, I mean, I have a terrific endo and his support and the clinic that I go to, the diabetes educator I've been going to there. I've even been going to a nutritionist. That's all taken care of . . . I'm almost afraid he [the endocrinologist] might do the test again and say, "You might be type 1 given how high your A1C is." I always thought, "At least that way I don't have to feel that I brought this on myself."

Mary's comment about "bringing it on herself" is not an uncommon feeling among people with type 2 diabetes. Situations that involve food, in particular, evidence this idea of a lack of willpower. For people with diabetes, holiday gatherings and dining out often become a struggle between wanting to act *normal* and following their therapies in order to avoid complications of the disease. Peel, Parry, Douglas, and Lawton (2005) examine dietary management talk in terms of how dietary *cheating* is accounted for in order to maintain a compliant identity. This idea of cheating, whether on holidays or any other day, is prevalent in online patient spaces as well. Some community members take offense at the use of the word at all:

> I eat moderately low carb but when I go out I usually eat more carbs because I'm a vegetarian and the food available in your typical restaurant is pasta. I don't consider this cheating. I bolus for it and sometimes it works, sometimes it doesn't. I don't feel guilty about this, but don't do it often. I think the whole "guilt" and "cheating" idea is infantile and self-defeating.

Other people write about cheating as a kind of confessional, sharing sentiments such as "I'm cheating on the diet. (Just cheating in general!)." Much of the anxiety expressed by these individuals comes from public perceptions and discourse surrounding diabetes, but these perceptions exist within the online diabetic community as well and periodically surface as arguments about which type of the disease (type 1 or 2) is worse. Referring to an article in the *Chicago Tribune* (Deardorff, 2010) about this and other efforts to change the names of type 1 and type 2 diabetes, a commenter in the TuDiabetes community with type 2 declared,

> I resent the fact that it was basically just another type 2 bashing article. I'm
> sick and tired of hearing about how it's all our fault we have diabetes and that
> all we have to do is diet and exercise our way into a cure.

Another recent example of this argument took place around a petition that two women who have sons with type 1 posted on an online petition platform, Change.org. In the petition they state: "Our sons face this life-threatening disease with strength, courage and perseverance despite being subjected on a daily basis to ignorance and misconceptions. It is with their future in mind that we file this petition to bring clarity to two very different diseases—Type 1 and Type 2 Diabetes." The petition asks decision makers at the ADA (American Diabetes Association), NIH (National Institutes of Health), and IDF (International Diabetes Federation) to revise the names of both type 1 and type 2 diabetes to more accurately reflect the nature of each disease. Many people with type 1 and their family members posted comments to the petition on the Change.org website, such as this person with type 1:

> This is important to me because when I tell people I have diabetes they
> always think of type 2 and they don't think it is as serious as it is, and they
> think that I got it from eating a lot of junk food, and sweets. It upsets me
> because I never did, and I still don't. (Berman, 2013, Supporters section)

In the discourses of diabetes, the certainty of numbers is, as we see, articulated with morality. In other words, certain numbers should lead to certain *good* actions. Aristotle argued that such practical wisdom, or phronesis, allows us to pursue a goal, but virtue tells us how to pursue it (Warne, 2006). According to Aristotle, phronesis was a "habit of attentiveness that makes the resources of one's past experiences flexibly available to one and, at the same time, allows the present situation to 'unconceal' its own particular significance" (Dunne, 1993, p. 305). In diabetes self-management, such practical wisdom would lead to an excellent decision and be the end result of control. If a person's blood sugar were too high, the excellent decision would be to take action that results in lowering the blood sugar number. As such, action is not contextualized but is assumed to be tied to a definition of what is right: a definition intertwined with the biomedical definition of compliance and narratives of progress. When a person tests her blood sugar level at home, for example, she may find that one day these values are 100, 160, 149, and 162 mg/dL. The next day the numbers may be 216, 200, 198, and 114 mg/dL. And so on. As people with diabetes go through each day, they make dozens of possibly *excellent decisions* in relation to these numbers. Let's say a person tests his blood sugar and it is 180 mg/dL—higher than it should be. The actions that people with diabetes take to *correct* these numbers are designed to *reset* the body and put it back into a state of homeostasis—a state in which blood glucose and insulin are in balance. The person with the 180 mg/dL might ask himself: Do I do nothing to try to get the number lower? Do I take a shot of insulin? Do I exercise? The excellent, ethical decision would be to take action that results in lowering high blood sugar numbers. And yet, because diabetes is a permanently liminal state, the excellent decision is always a moving target. Because the equation used to balance medicine/insulin with the amount of carbohydrate eaten is not guaranteed to work, intent is only part of the equation.

NARRATIVES OF PROGRESS AND THE HISTORY OF DIABETES TECHNOLOGIES

Along with surveillance, numbers, and identities, the ethical action of controlling blood sugar is articulated with the theme of progress in diabetes discourse and texts. Within the terministic screen of compliance, the question becomes: How do I progress from uncontrolled/noncompliant/unknowledgeable/bad to an expert identity (a person with specialized knowledge that takes actions to control blood sugar levels) and an improved body (a body that is kept within a targeted blood sugar range)? In diabetes, this theme begins as the story of insulin. Like other medications, insulin is a technological innovation, and, as such, the narrative becomes one of technological progress. This progress is embedded in ideas about technological development as evolutionary in nature, much like Darwin's idea of continuity in our evolution, which highlights our similarities to animals.[15] Phyletic gradualism similarly argues that evolutionary change is marked by a pattern of smooth and continuous

---

15. Burke (1966) argued that Darwin stressed the idea of continuity in our evolution and highlights our similarities to animals. Theologians, on the other hand, focus on our discontinuity to animals and readjust our continuity to be with other humans and God (p. 50).

change in the fossil record.[16] Similar "progress" models are apparent in the natural sciences and the social sciences. Kuhn (1962) argues that, prior to his work, historians of science represented the development of scientific theory as a gradual process.[17] Both cultural anthropology and archaeology use Sahlins and Service's (1960) categories of band, tribe, chiefdom, and state as a framework for understanding various societies. These distinctions use political, social, and economic characteristics of increasing complexity that determine which category a society falls within. Whereas bands tend to be kin-based groups (that is, all members of the group are related to each other by kinship or marriage ties), chiefdoms are composed of different groups of people who are organized into a hierarchical social system, for example.

Exemplary of the fact that the narrative of diabetes is bound to the narrative of technological progress is the attention Michael Bliss pays to the technology of insulin in his 2007 book. Granted, the book specifically focuses on the discovery of insulin, but diabetes has been recognized for more than two thousand years. Insulin has existed for approximately one hundred years. In the book, Bliss spends a mere 20 or so pages on what he calls "a long prelude" (p. 20) to the discovery, vividly describing what was in store for people with diabetes before insulin was available. In his historical text, Bliss articulates the disease with this technology in a way that mirrors both public and medical narrations of the disease. People with type 1 diabetes (particularly children) traditionally are represented as victims, like Julia Roberts's movie character, while people with type 2 are often seen as villains—people not willing to take care of themselves. Doctors are heroes discovering cures. But technology is an even bigger hero, and the tale of technological progress is particularly important in diabetes care because insulin changed the trajectory of the disease. As Feudtner (2003) tells it,

> Perhaps no story of medical progress, though, has been more influenced by this technology ethos than the history of diabetes. Stories of insulin have served various needs while reinforcing deeply held beliefs of twentieth century Americans. A parable of salvation, the tale of diabetic deliverance has

---

16. See Eldredge and Gould (1972) for an alternative theory of punctuated equilibrium that suggests that while evolution has long periods of evolutionary stability, these periods are marked by instances of branching evolution, a process in which a species splits into smaller groups, which leads to an evolutionary adaptive process because greater diversity is created.

17. Kuhn also says that while this is the path of *normal* science, sometimes anomalies occur that cannot be explained by such a gradual process. (Normal science produces three types of research: research that determines specific factual details within the theory, research that matches theory to observations, and research that clarifies problems in an existing paradigm.)

spoken to the imagination of doctors and laypeople alike, serving as a potent and often cited symbol of scientific progress and the prospect of human mastery over disease. One of the most impressive stories about modern medical miracles, the tale of insulin saving diabetics has legitimized the prestige and power that Americans have invested in scientific medicine and its technical wizardry. (pp. 9–10)

The discovery of insulin, described as "one of the most dramatic events in the history of the treatment of the disease" (2007, p. 11), occurred at the University of Toronto in 1921. In his well-researched text, Bliss explains that in the late in the nineteenth century, scientists knew there was a connection between the pancreas and diabetes, a connection further narrowed down to the islets of Langerhans, a part of the pancreas. In the early 1900s, researchers tried unsuccessfully to find and extract the active ingredient from the islets of Langerhans. While reading a paper on the subject in 1920, Canadian surgeon Frederick Banting had an idea: He wanted to isolate and study the islets of Langerhans hormone by stopping the pancreas from working but keeping the islets of Langerhans going. He presented this idea to John J. R. Macleod, the head of the department of physiology at the University of Toronto. MacLeod initially derided the idea, but he eventually gave Banting lab space, 10 laboratory dogs, and a medical student assistant, Charles Best, to research his idea. By August of 1921, Banting and Best had conclusive results that when they gave the material extracted from the islets of Langerhans (called *insulin,* from the Latin for *island*) to dogs with diabetes, the dogs' high blood sugar levels came down. After replicating the experiment several times with similar results and working to purify the insulin, Banting was confident enough to try it in an experiment on a human: a 14-year-old boy dying of diabetes. The injection lowered the boy's blood sugar. Banting and Best published their first paper on the discovery a month later, in February 1922. In 1923, Banting and Macleod were awarded the Nobel Prize for their discovery.

The narrative of technological and scientific wonder that unfolds in Bliss's book is apparent in news headlines and articles of the time. A 1923 headline in *The New York Times* trumpeted "Diabetes, Dread Disease, Yields to New Gland Cure." The article stated that, "one by one, the implacable enemies of man, the disease which seek his destruction, are overcome by science" (Collins, 1923, p. 12). A 1922 article in the same paper characterized Dr. Banting as one of the heroes, saying that he was "applauded as he told how the curative agent was worked out from knowledge that the interstitial cells of the pancreatic gland were the main factor in assimilation of sugar" (*The New York Times,* 1922, p. 9). A 1935 *New York Times* headline also evoked the positive nature of scientific and technological progress and the symbolism of scientists and physicians as authorities: "Urge More Use of Insulin: Experts Find that Fear Now Blocks the Cure of Diabetes."

Even though the narrative of technological progress in diabetes is firmly articulated with the discovery of insulin, the history of technology and diabetes does not stop with the discovery of the hormone. As insulin pump technologies become more complex, inhalable versions of insulin are created, and rumors of stem cell replacement therapy surface in both scientific journals and in online patient forum discussions; contemporary discourses of diabetes still privilege a narrative of technological progress. Less heralded than these *miraculous* technologies, but equally important, are the surveillance technologies of diabetes, particularly the home blood glucose testing meter. These technologies articulate with contemporary diabetes care and discourse that involves medication, diet, and exercise. In the lived experience of the disease, these articulations are not always positive, as the excerpts from my focus group participants express.

> GRACE: And now I have a pump on me 24/7, which means I always have that reminder, so I'm always thinking about it. And I also had a Dexcom for a while. So I was CONSTANTLY looking at that thing. I'm like, "Oh my god." And my family would say, "Oh, it must be so much easier," and I'd go, "No, it's not." It's a constant reminder. I'm constantly thinking and checking and looking.
>
> CONNIE: That's what I find now. All the things we have at our fingertips that are keeping us up to date. Like back in the, like before we got blood meters, I just tested my urine and I gave one shot a day and I did fine.

Even so, the hope for better technology and the hope for a cure remain strong motifs in discourses surrounding diabetes. This discourse is most apparent on the Juvenile Diabetes Research Foundation's (JDRF) website and related materials. One technological initiative discussed on the JDRF website is the artificial pancreas, a technology that would automatically control a person's blood glucose level in a manner similar to the way a healthy pancreas does. While a person could still make insulin-dosing adjustments, the artificial pancreas is a system designed to calculate how much insulin a pump delivers based on readings from a CGM. Such a system requires little or no input from the user. According to the JDRF website and an article in *Diabetes Forecast* (Berg, 2014), the technology will make managing type 1 easier and less of a burden for individuals with the disease. JDRF also advertises its research and advocacy efforts for the technology as moving from type 1 to a nation of "Type None" (JDRF, 2016, About JDRF section), implying if not a cure then the eradication of the disease.

This cure discourse is also apparent in the talk and texts produced by people with the disease. A 2001 post by diabetic blogger Scott Hanselman said, for example,

> I imagine a world of true digital convergence—assuming that I won't be cured of diabetes by some biological means in my lifetime—an implanted pump and glucose sensor, an advanced artificial pancreas. A closed system for diabetics that automatically senses sugar levels and delivers insulin has been the diabetics' holy grail for years. But with the advent of wireless technology and the Internet, my already optimistic vision has brightened. If I had an implanted device with wireless capabilities, it could be in constant contact with my doctor. (Hanselman, 2014, para. 35)

NARRATIVES OF PROGRESS AND DIABETES EDUCATIONAL TEXTS

The historical connection between diabetes and technology generates articulations to progress that extend beyond technology to include progress to expert identities and improved bodies, which become evidence of patient agency. Texts used to educate and inform people with diabetes are technological instruments as well, and just as blood glucose meters make blood sugar readings visible, these texts make the articulation between the constellation of compliance, agency, control, surveillance, identities, and morality visible. The narratives in these texts are articulated with the technological narrative of progress, but here they also align with medical goals of achieving control and expert, autonomous patients. The process of getting blood sugar under control is often presented in diabetic educational materials as a journey.[18] A second visual metaphor is the ladder.

The journey for control is one from the starting point of being an uninformed patient to the end point of being an expert on diabetes, which assumes that there is an end and that progress has been made in getting to that end. These narratives share much with the monomyth, or hero's journey (Campbell, 2008), in which the hero ventures from the everyday world into a world

---

18. Examples include Sanofi's program Our Diabetes Journey—For Parents and Kids and Merck's Journey for Control® program. See the Sanofi-Aventis website at www.a1cchampions.com/about-a1c-champions/our-diabetes-journey.aspx and Merck's website at www.journeyforcontrol.com.

of supernatural wonder. The hero encounters foes along the way but eventually returns to bestow a boon (i.e., a holy grail) on her community. In the texts examined for this project, progress is similarly defined as movement/advancement toward a goal. Both the ADA and Joslin websites draw more subtly on a journey metaphor with the use of the phrase *getting started*. The following text is from a page on the Joslin Diabetes Center's website called Diabetes and Scheduling: Starting a Routine.

Getting Started

In order to implement a routine when you have diabetes, it's first important to gain a good understanding of what major factors influence blood glucose levels, so you can keep them in mind while building your routine. Some major factors that influence blood glucose levels include:

- food/meals
- physical activity
- diabetes medications and/or insulin[19]

Text from the ADA's Blood Glucose Control web page also uses the phrase *getting started* to explain that a person does not need to figure these things out on his own.

Whatever method you choose, your health care team (your doctor, dietitian, diabetes educator, and other health care professionals) should spend a lot of time teaching you about it. Your team will help you make guidelines for how much insulin to take and when. You will also come up with guidelines for eating and exercising. These guidelines may change several times as you test them out.[20]

The journey motif is also embedded in the Conversation Maps that a CDE who was interviewed for this study uses in her group educational sessions.[21] The Conversation Maps use a similar progress narrative in relation to seeing life with the disease as a journey. The Conversation Map Program includes

19. Copyright © 2016 by Joslin Diabetes Center. All rights reserved. Reprinted with permission from www.joslin.org.

20. Copyright © 2013–2015 American Diabetes Association. From: www.diabetes.org. Reprinted with permission from the American Diabetes Association.

21. The Conversation Map program tools and materials are intellectual property created and owned by Healthy Interactions in collaboration with the American Diabetes Association (ADA) and sponsored by Merck.

five maps. People attending a group educational session sit around the map and play a game that is somewhat similar to Hasbro's board game The Game of Life: They take turns and move along a path that winds its way from the beginning of the game to the end. In the first map, the diabetes overview, the journey is taken by car. In the second, which focuses on healthy eating, the journey is a walk through a market. The third map's journey is facilitated by hot-air balloons, and the fourth map involves a walk across a bridge. The fifth map, which targets people with gestational diabetes, portrays the journey as a walk through a garden.

Even outside of a regular education group session, Daisy, the CDE, relies on this journey metaphor. During her interview she even led me through a description of how she used the map as a journey.

> When they do that on the map over here, it will encourage people to get up, walk around. They say put it on a table, but of course here we have no table. So right here we start with definition. They suggest you have someone read it. Sometimes people get funny about reading things in front of other people—school-type things. So I will say, "Would anybody like to?" If they don't, that's all right, too. Then it says, "Remember, you're in the driver's seat," so it's showing the car and then people who are helpers. But the people in the car have the diabetes. Then we talk about what are the myths. What kinds of things have you heard about diabetes? We have a list of cards that we hand out that I have over there in my little pouch. We'll say, "Read yours." Then, "What do you think? Is that a myth or a fact?" Then we'll discuss it. If someone gets it wrong, we'll say, "You know, a lot of people feel that way, and that's why we will want to talk about it." [. . .]
>
> LA: Are all the cards myths? Or some are facts?[22]
> DAISY: Yeah. Eating too much sugar causes diabetes. You can catch diabetes from somebody else. People with diabetes are more likely to get colds and other illnesses. That is true. But I added some more to it, and I have some more over there. Blood glucose monitoring can help you manage your diabetes—yes. Smoking increases the risk—yes. You're in charge of managing—yes. You could lower high blood glucose with high fiber foods—yes. Your body needs carbohydrates for energy—yes. So there is a mixture. That's part of what you do there.

---

22. In the interview, excerpts from "LA" refer to the author.

We continued with a short discussion of administrative details and a digression about a common acquaintance. Then, to get the conversation back on track, I said: "Let's move on." Daisy replied, "That's exactly right; let's move on." As this exchange shows, the journey narrative can be powerful: I easily fell in step with the narrative in this particular interview process, which was evident from my use of the phrase *let's move on*.

As concepts that help people understand things outside of their own direct experience (Lakoff & Johnson, 1980), metaphors get mapped from a source domain of experience to another idea in a target domain. For example, in the metaphor *disease is a war,* the source domain is *war* and the target domain is *disease.* By making this connection, the speaker creates the idea of disease for his or her audience as something that must be fought against and is possible to win against. The journey metaphor emphasizes the singularity of patient identity by emphasizing diabetes as a personal odyssey or pilgrimage. The car metaphor that Daisy uses when she references the images on the maps is related to using a journey metaphor of living with diabetes as well mapping onto what Judy Segal (2005) points out to be one of the primary metaphors used in medical discourse—that of the body as a machine. This metaphor has led to people using this language in self-descriptions, such as being "wound up" like a clock or "worn out" like an old furnace (Segal, 2005, p. 121). Similarly, people with diabetes use car language to talk about episodes of low blood sugar as *crashing* or being *in the driver's seat* with diabetes, as a parent of a child with diabetes describes her son's work when he is away from home: "I'd say he does 90 percent of the work when he and I are apart. When he's home, we're definitely a team. He makes decisions, I make decisions, we make decisions together. When he's at school or elsewhere, he's in the driver's seat."

This idea of being in the driver's seat gives a somewhat mixed message. On the one hand, the person is driving from one place to another. As such, the metaphor articulates the idea of the agency and expertise being the boon acquired at the end of a journey. At the same time, by being the driver (i.e., the person in control of a car), the metaphor takes on nuances of the metaphor of the body as machine, a metaphor entrenched in biomedicine (Segal, 2005), and leads to practices in which patients are seen as being able to be repaired and have their so-called parts replaced. However, in this chronic illness context, being in the driver's seat can also be articulated to the home hobbyist or the user-producers Kimball discusses (2006). This person takes care of her own repairs, tinkering and adjusting as needed.

The ladder, another image used to indicate progress, is part of a form called My Plan to Take Charge which was developed and is used by a group of pharmacists for group diabetes educational appointments. The form has spaces for the participant to write down the answers to six questions:

1. Is there anything I would like to do to improve my health?
2. What is *one* step I can take to make this improvement?
3. How will I know if I have accomplished my goal?
4. What conditions would have to exist in order to meet my goal?
5. Am I dependent on anyone else to achieve my goal?
6. On a scale of 1–10, how likely am I to accomplish my goal?

These questions are followed by the image of a ladder. Beside the bottom step are the words "0 not sure at all." At the fifth step are the words "5 somewhat sure," and at the top of the ladder is "10 very sure." The ladder functions as a spatial metaphor. In such a metaphor, up is associated with good and down with bad. On the ladder, a person on the top step is confident that she can be in control. The person on the bottom step is unsure and out of control. To be in control, she must make progress up the ladder. Ladders similarly evoke end-like visions, such as that of Maslow's (2015) hierarchy of needs, which is visualized as a pyramid with self-actualization at the top. Inherent in images like ladders and pyramids is Burke's (1950) hierarchic principle. This principle is not merely the relation of higher to lower but includes the tendency to view the top as the best position, which allows for scapegoats to be created. Burke (1950) explains:

> And as the principle of *any* hierarchy involves the possibility of reversing highest and lowest, so the moralizing of status makes for a revolutionary kind of expression, the scapegoat. The scapegoat is dialectically appealing, since it combines in one figure contrary principles of identification and alienation. And by splitting the hierarchic principle into factions, it becomes ritually gratifying; for each faction can then use the other as *katharma,* the unclean vessel upon which can be loaded the dyslogistic burdens of a vocabulary. . . . (pp. 140–41)

The articulation of control, surveillance, subjectivities of spoiled identities, and narratives and metaphors of progress align with the diminished definition of patient agency as a means-to-an-end equation. The intention of this first chapter has been to reveal these articulations in order to *re-articulate* agency as something enacted through the temporary articulations that people with chronic illnesses make to knowledge, subjectivities, and discourses. *Re-articulating* agency from the perspective of medical rhetoric and its related fields can redirect our terministic screen (Burke, 1966), which plays a significant part in determining what we can see and say about agency. To make this shift, the following chapters offer a series of re-articulations to show that agency is flexible and multiplicitous. To begin to articulate bodies and language requires "spatializ[ing] the world to accommodate them" (Stormer, 2004, p. 263). In this project, bodies and language are spatialized through what is described as the liminal spaces of group appointments and online patient communities. Rhetorical work, including the enactment of agency, of people with diabetes is increasingly being conducted in spaces that are more and more uncertain, ambiguous, and fluid than the one-on-one patient-doctor appointment. In these liminal spaces of contemporary medicine, the unstable attachments between agency, liminal spaces, multiple types of knowledge, multiple subjectivities, and multiple performances of professional identities are made visible.

CHAPTER 2

Liminal Spaces

Counter Narratives and Writing as Social Action

> We are in the epoch of simultaneity: we are in the epoch of juxtaposition,
> the epoch of the near and far, of the side-by-side, of the dispersed. We are at
> a moment, I believe, when our experience of the world is less that of a long
> life developing through time than that of a network that connects points and
> intersects with its own skein.
>
> —M. Foucault, "Of Other Spaces, Heterotopias"

LIMINAL SPACES

Spaces used for medical care have historically varied in ways that suggest juxtaposition more than simultaneity. As industrialization occurred, medicine, once practiced at the patient's bedside, began to shift from patients' homes to both hospitals and doctors' offices. Foucault (1994), focusing on the reorganization of knowledge at the end of the eighteenth century in the form of the space of the "clinic" (teaching hospitals), traces these changes in nineteenth-century France. Prior to this time, hospitals existed, but they were typically occupied by the poor or soldiers and cared for by "inadequately trained doctors and experienced quacks" (Foucault, 1994, p. 66). America followed a similar timeline to France in this change: The first hospital that catered to the sick and the poor was established in 1751 in Philadelphia. New York Hospital was established about twenty years later and Massachusetts General Hospital in 1811 (Porter, 1999).[1]

Medical care has also been relegated to the traditional doctor visit, a visit Segal (2005) describes as the central encounter in health care. Think back to Tom, whom we met in the introduction. When he goes to the doctor, he sits

---

1. The merger of scientific and medical education as well as technological advances in surgery in the nineteenth century also impacted medical practices (Porter, 1999).

in the waiting room. When the door opens to the back, the nurse takes Tom to the digital scale to record his weight then leads him back to an exam room to take his blood pressure and take his pulse. Stationing herself in front of the computer screen in the room, she begins to ask a list of questions.

1. Do you smoke? Any alcohol?
2. How many times do you exercise each week?
3. Do you need any prescriptions filled?

Finishing her tasks, the nurse leaves the room with Tom's blood glucose meter in order to download and print out the test results. She tells Tom that the doctor will be in soon. In the meantime, Tom reads the fliers on the wall about flu shots and checks the list of questions he brought for this particular visit. When the doctor enters, he discusses the downloaded blood test results with Tom. He checks Tom's heartbeat, hands, and feet and writes up orders for lab work for an A1C test and kidney function analysis. When the doctor leaves, the phlebotomist comes in to draw blood and then sends Tom on his way.

Time is an important factor in such spaces. As this hypothetical scenario suggests, in traditional office visits a single patient interacts with doctors, nurses, medical assistants, and office staff one-on-one in a manner that stresses linear conceptions of time. Time is emphasized through insurance company rules as well. For example, the primary care physicians that work in the practices associated with my university's teaching hospital have 15 minutes to spend with each patient. Specialists, like endocrinologists, are allotted 20 or 30 minutes. Time and timing are important aspects of the disease itself, too. Diabetes is progressive, so the longer a person has the disease the more likely it is for a diabetic to develop complications such as neuropathy, which often causes numbness or pain in the feet; kidney problems and possibly kidney failure; and cardiovascular disease, for example. Timing is just as important if a person takes any form of medication, such as oral agents like Metformin or injectable insulin. The actions of these medications have arcs, so it is critical to time these arcs with food to try to stabilize, or normalize, blood sugar levels.

But space is important as well. In such clinical encounters things happen in a sequence of spaces: the waiting room, the "outer chamber" with a nurse or medical assistant, and finally the private exam room with the doctor. Patients must present evidence of insurance and sign waivers before the medical personnel can touch their bodies to monitor the status of their health. Even with the current emphasis on patient–centered care and shared decision making, this sequence of spaces continues to emphasize medical authority: Patients must be invited back to the area where this work is performed, as Tom was in the preceding scenario, and must wait to be seen by the doctor.[2] In diabetes care, these encounters have changed little since insulin was discovered in 1922. Feudtner (2003) describes a visit to the Joslin Diabetes Clinic in the mid-1920s:

> Up the steps and through the door, the patients—if they had heeded instructions and come prepared—left a bottle of their urine, neatly labeled, in the small laboratory room that was immediately to their left. Farther up the hall they came to the room where several secretaries kept the clinic in motion. After registering, the patients would ascend the next flight of stairs to the second floor and take a seat in the large hallway that served as the waiting room. . . . Sitting in the hallway, those patients who were devotees of Joslin's *Manual* may have thumbed through their personal notebooks, preparing to "show it to [their] physician at each visit." In these booklets, Joslin advised, "all questions about symptoms and diet which have arisen since the former visit should be neatly set down, with space left for an answer to each question. (pp. 92–93)

Spaces other than the clinic are just as important in the circumstance of chronic illness. Corbin and Strauss (1988) have theorized the work of chronic illness outside of clinical spaces as a process that involves an interaction between the physical progression of the disease, everyday life work (work in domestic spaces that is not related to caring for a disease), and biographical work. They rightly argue that self-caring for a chronic illness is work, but their metaphor of a trajectory (the path that a moving object follows through space as a function of time) and progression still prioritize time and equate work to performing tasks—two facts that keep this sense of work embedded in compliance. This process also keeps the work done in the two spheres distinct, and yet as Tom's statement at the opening of this book makes clear, people with chronic illnesses engage in medical work at home.

Because spaces are ideological, lived, and subjective (Lefebvre, 1991),[3] maintaining the binary distinction between clinic and home reinforces cul-

---

2. Of course, many doctors knock on the door before entering the exam room a patient is in, but just as often, they enter the room before the patient gives any response inviting the doctor in.

3. Until the twentieth century, space was subordinate to time, but Foucault (1984a) argued that we now live in an epoch of space, an assertion that is supported by the spatial turn a variety of disciplines have taken. Foucault (1984a) argued that the history of space in Western culture has been one that began in Medieval times and is what he calls "a hierarchic ensemble of places" (para. 2). He gives examples such as sacred and profane places and urban and rural places. He argued that this hierarchy of oppositions is a space of emplacement. In other words,

tural assumptions about doctors and patients based on the spheres they are expected to inhabit, much as cultural assumptions about gender are influenced by space (see Kerber, 1988). A current metaphor for the health care system, the medical neighborhood, attempts to challenge some of these assumptions by moving the home into the clinic, so to speak. In one illustration of this neighborhood, the patient-centered medical home (where patients receive care and where their information is housed) is in the center.[4] The neighbors surrounding this home include pharmacists, a hospital, medical specialists, insurance companies, primary care physicians, and community social services. As anyone going to multiple doctors can attest to, in the past (particularly before the use of electronic medical records), physicians have often relied on patients to get information from other sources back to them. The intent of the medical neighborhood model is to better coordinate care and communicate with each other rather than relying on patients to "serve as the main conduit of information between the clinicians they see" (AHRQ, 2011, p. 1). Instead, the goals are to coordinate care between a variety of care providers (AHRQ, 2011). For instance, specialists should let primary care physicians know what type of routine care the patient needs with regard to the specialized treatment the patient is receiving (such as follow-up care after a surgery). Primary care doctors should make referrals to specialists and give these specialists any clinical data about a patient that the specialist may need, and hospitals should inform primary care physicians about any hospital visits of their patients. These activities ensure that when a patient has been in the hospital the person's primary care physician is notified, for example.

Although placing the home in the clinical neighborhood could potentially challenge cultural assumptions about the actors in these two distinct spaces, the ideology of this neighborhood continues to emphasize order, time, rationality, and medical authority. At the same time, it marginalizes patients that make use of the neighborhood in two ways. They are marginalized by the lack of images of people among the buildings in this neighborhood, an omission

---

it involves the location of something. Social theory in particular has repositioned ideas about space as something that exists a priori to something that is produced. As put by Warf (2009), "Location, in short, has become increasingly a matter of production and negotiation rather than being given a priori" (p. 69). Both Foucault and Lefebvre were instrumental in drawing this attention to space. For an excellent introduction to other spatial scholars, see *Key Thinkers on Space and Place,* edited by Phil Hubbard, Rob Kitchin, and Gill Valentine (2004).

4. The patient-centered medical home is a health care initiative that focuses on coordinating care between specialists, primary care doctors, and hospitals. The *home* is a term coined in the literature by Fisher (2008) in a description of barriers associated with medical homes working successfully. Pham (2010) and the American College of Physicians, in a position paper (ACP 2010), further develop the idea of the medical neighborhood. The illustration I describe can be accessed at: www.pcpcc.org/event/2014/08/2014-mid-atlantic-medical-neighborhood-forum.

that emphasizes coordinating information, as opposed to surveilling bodies. The absence of patients' homes in the medical neighborhood also marginalizes the self-monitoring people with diabetes do even though this self-monitoring is a critical aspect of the information flow providers are trying to coordinate. In the medical neighborhood, the conversation about organizing care is exclusive to the activities of medical providers even though the flow of information from the patient is the first step in helping to coordinate care as well as treatment decisions. This absence suggests that care is a one-way activity and, rather than adding to the collective work of the neighborhood, patients are end users of the products and interventions developed for them by the members of this neighborhood.

The focus of this model, therefore, remains on the clinicians and institutions and the work they do. Aside from Keränen's (2007) and Owen's (2009) research, most of the literature in medical rhetoric leaves the patient out of the work that goes on *within* health care as well. Much of the scholarship produced by Catherine Schryer and her team, for example, focuses on education and professionalization issues in medical discourse. McCarthy's (1991) work with the *Diagnostic and Statistical Manual of Mental Disorders* (DSM) is another example: She looks at the collaborative process medical professionals undertook to revise the DSM-III to the DSM-IV. Other work has focused on investigations of genres used by employees in medical workplaces.[5]

The result of these absences is that the work of people with diabetes remains invisible and undervalued. This work is not just the daily monitoring and clinical tasks of testing blood sugar levels and taking medication, people with diabetes are also acting as symbolic analysts, processing information and symbols. And yet, even when bodies are present in clinical spaces, they are often regarded only as recorders of information. In an exam room this is clear. The doctor or medical assistant sits behind a computer screen or stands before the patient. The patient sits or reclines on the exam table as an object of study and hands his meter over to a medical assistant to download and print out his blood sugar numbers. Many if not most blood glucose meters on the market store data (i.e., the results from blood sugar tests). The amount varies, but typically meters can store at least 30 days of results. Both people with diabetes and their doctors can download these data to look at trends. These trends, in turn, might indicate a need for changes in diabetes treatment. If, for example, Tom took his meter in to his doctor appointment, the doctor might download

---

5. See Berkenkotter and Ravotas (1997); Popham (2005); Popham & Graham (2008); Schryer (1993) and (1994); and Schryer and Spoel, (2005). Some work in feminist technical communication scholarship (see Koerber, 2006 and 2013; Seigel, 2014) does position patients within the medical system as well.

the results and find that Tom always has very high blood sugar from 4 a.m. to 6 a.m. Tom and his doctor would talk about adjusting the amount of insulin his pump delivers to him during those hours. Sheri, one of my focus group participants, describes this interaction this way:

> In the beginning I used to really monitor everything in great detail. I used an Excel spreadsheet and I kept a detail of that. I don't have a CGM or anything like that. But now, when I really want to keep a log of things, I use my Bayer Contour USB meter, which automatically logs everything . . . it charts things . . . it just keeps record of that and I can plug it into my doctor's computer if she really wants to look at those numbers and such.

If we think about agency as a possession—a package of knowledge that can simply be transferred from one person to the next—this exchange of blood sugar numbers might seem agential on the surface. In the documentary *The Art of the Possible,* an exchange of information from doctor to patient is certainly portrayed as such. In the movie, which narrates the efforts in children's cancer treatment at the University of Texas MD Anderson Cancer Center in Houston, Texas, a scene shows Dr. Peter Anderson interacting with a patient. In this interaction, Anderson hands the patient a flash drive loaded with the patient's medical information. According to Anderson, this action gives the patient a sense of ownership and empowerment. But is this sensibility reverse engineered when a patient with diabetes gives her doctor her meter? Does the patient feel ownership of her information or does the doctor? The text on one of the ADA's web pages might help answer these questions. The following is part of the Blood Glucose Control page under the heading "What do my results mean?"

> When you finish the blood glucose check, write down your results and review them to see how food, activity and stress affect your blood glucose. Take a close look at your blood glucose record to see if your level is too high or too low several days in a row at about the same time. If the same thing keeps happening, it might be time to change your plan. Work with your doctor or diabetes educator to learn what your results mean for you. This takes time. Ask your doctor or nurse if you should report results out of a certain range at once by phone.[6]

---

6. Copyright © 2013–2015 American Diabetes Association. From www.diabetes.org. Reprinted with permission from the American Diabetes Association.

Pomerantz and Rintel (2004) have suggested that patients and providers approach medical encounters with certain assumptions about their positions and the roles of each other. Their study reports that when communicating test results to patients, if doctors provide numerical readings without providing interpretations, they cast the patient as an independent expert. When they communicate results with only an interpretation of the results, the doctor is assuming a more paternalistic role. Here, the person with diabetes is advised to read, record, and note patterns, but then to "work with your doctor or diabetes educator to learn what your results mean for you." The phrase "work with" implies that the person with diabetes is taking an active role in the conversations and decisions being made about the treatment plan, and is, in fact, a partner in this relationship. However, the person with diabetes does not assign meaning to the blood sugar patterns that emerge. The provider interprets the patterns and gives meaning to these patterns in the context of a clinical visit. As a recorder, the patient takes on the role as author of the body functions, but because no interpretation is required on his part, authorial authority is missing. In other words, the person remains invisible in the same way as the technicians at the engineering center in Winsor's (2003) research or a technical communicator writing a software manual who does not get a "byline" or credit for creating the documents.[7] Providing numerical readings without interpretation in this way also implies that the physician possesses the knowledge to make such interpretation on his own. The implication is that the doctor's office is where action, problem solving, and interpretation take place.[8] This assumption is prevalent in educational and informational materials produced for people with diabetes by a variety of institutions, corporations, and government agencies.

Replacing these assumptions with new ones that are more attuned to a relational definition of agency requires locating the person with diabetes *inside* medicine. In other words, although the treatment of diabetes may not be located in the body (Mol & Law, 2004), the body must be located within the space of work in which care occurs. We can see this work in less binary spaces than those of the home and the clinic. Two such spaces without such discrete boundaries between scientific ways of knowing the body and more private, personal ways of knowing the body are group appointments and online patient communities. In general, group appointments follow the same

---

7. It is interesting to note that with the move to finding computer technical support help through online forums, this may be changing in the general field of technical communication.

8. With the advent of software programs associated with continuous glucose monitoring systems and blood glucose meters, people with diabetes have new opportunities to read and analyze blood sugar trends by themselves, outside of the doctor visit.

format as medical doctor visits—those including one patient and one provider.[9] Although, no single definition for a group medical/educational visit exists, one reason they emerged was as a way for physicians to better manage their time by seeing a number of patients collectively in one appointment (Noffsinger & Scott, 2000). The appointments themselves are usually planned as an extended medical appointment with an added component of a behavioral health professional (counselor, nurse, or educator). The appointments are typically facilitated by the physician and the other specialist. Medical assistants also provide direct care such as taking blood pressures, testing blood sugar levels, and negotiating charts and other paperwork. In diabetes care, group educational appointments have also emerged. These appointments specifically focus on having patients discuss how to manage their disease and learn self-care behaviors from each other as well as from the medical professional facilitating the session. In shared appointments, a doctor, a certified diabetes educator, a pharmacist, or a nurse might give a short talk about how to recognize symptoms of low blood sugar. A nutritionist might lead the group on a grocery store tour to talk about how to read food labels, or a diabetes educator might employ a Conversation Map[10] to generate discussion among patients in a shared appointment. Discussions between the patients in the class are encouraged as well. These interactions add an element of surprise to the classes; the facilitator has a plan but the interactions between the diabetics in the room create a fluid environment in which articulations are open to shifts.

Online patient communities are also social spaces in which people with diabetes and their family members interact. A number of online diabetes patient communities moderated by health care organizations exist, but TuDiabetes is a grassroots organization that grew out of the Diabetes Hands Founda-

---

9. In the last decade, group appointments have been found to be a feasible (and cost-effective) way to deliver education. Nearly 70 percent of the patients cited the benefit of self-care education (McInaney, 2000). In a study specifically centered on diabetes care, Mehl-Madrona (2010) presented early-phase clinical investigations focusing on efforts at improving care for Native Americans and found that shared, collaborative care was more helpful than group care or individualized care alone. Other entities pursuing group appointments include Harvard Vanguard Medical Associates, which hosts more than 30 shared medical appointments at six of its 21 locations (McCarthy, 2010); the Cincinnati VA Medical Center (S. Mohn, personal communication, October 3, 2010); the Northern Kentucky Health Department (Northern Kentucky Health Department staff, personal communication, July 10, 2010); the YMCA through a partnership with UnitedHealthcare (A. Poetker, personal communication, August 10, 2010); and several pharmacies in the Cincinnati area (N. Kunze, personal communication, November 9, 2010).

10. Created and owned by Healthy Interactions, in collaboration with the American Diabetes Association (ADA), and sponsored by Merck.

tion, which was started by Manny Hernandez in 2007.[11] The statistics posted on the website in January 2016 state that since that time there have been 47,500 topics posted; 40,700 new members; and 17,400 "likes." Members include people with type 1, type 2, type 1.5 (also known as LADA), and gestational diabetes as well as friends and family members of people with the disease. The TuDiabetes website, like all websites, is not exactly stable. It is as dynamic as the diabetic body—a body in constant flux seeking to find equilibrium. The site offers the ability to upload photos and videos as well as real-time chat and blogs along with its discussion boards. The membership and content are constantly changing: People take down old pictures and replace them with new ones as well as start new discussions every hour and add replies to others. When asked how often they visited the website, one of my interviewees responded, "Well, as one of the six volunteer administrators/forum moderators, I am on the site AT LEAST one hour a day. Most days, I check in every few hours and see how my assigned area (which varies by month) is going, spend 15–20 minutes reading over people's posts, and move on to the rest of my day."

Unlike traditional spaces of medical care, such dynamic spaces require a spatialized ontology that recognizes "spatiality as simultaneously a social product and a shaping force of social life" (Soja, 1989, p. 7). Like Foucault (1984a), Soja argues that the nineteenth century interest in history gives way to an interest in space in later centuries.[12] Of course, rhetoric itself has long been spatialized in both concrete and geographical terms.[13] Contemporary scholars also continue to spatialize the rhetorical situation in increasingly

---

11. The author is a member of the TuDiabetes online community.

12. Soja (1996), following the work of Lefebvre (1991), argued that the organization of space is a critical dimension of society and reflects social facts and influences social relations. In other words, he talked of power in terms of spatial justice, which links together social justice and space. Cintron (1998) talked about power and space in terms of "making," the processes by which people make their lives fit their environment and their environment fit their lives. Finally, in his discussion of strategies and tactics, de Certeau (1984) aligned strategy with control by administration and management entities. Tactics, on the other hand, live in the domain of the nonpowerful. Like Cintron's trope of making, tactics are adaptations to the environment.

13. Classical rhetors used spatial metaphors of a house or a building in their minds to try to organize and recollect appeals for their use. More contemporary conversations about space in rhetoric are largely driven by the concept of the rhetorical situation. These conversations were famously driven by the debate between Bitzer (1968) and Vatz (1973) that started close to half a century ago about the rhetorical situation. As scholars of rhetoric know, Bitzer (1968) defined the rhetorical situation as "the context in which speakers or writers create rhetorical discourse" (p. 1). In his view, the situation has to exist before discourse and rhetorical action do. Vatz (1973), on the other hand, argued that no situation is independent of the perception of the interpreter and discrete situations are largely mythical concepts in that they are rhetorically based and circumscribed (Vatz, 1973; 1981; 2006; and 2009). Rhetoric, in other words, defines the situation.

complex ways. Edbauer (2005), for instance, suggests that rhetorical theorists should shift "the lines of focus from *rhetorical situation* to *rhetorical ecologies*" (p. 9; emphasis in original). In a rhetorical ecology, speakers, texts, audiences, and exigencies do not pre-exist but are constituted through discursive activity. Drawing on Warner (2002), Biesecker (1989), and Phelps (1983), Edbauer (2005) argues that a notion of the rhetorical situation grounded in a "bordered, fixed space-location" (p. 9), cannot account for the fluidity and circulation of rhetoric.[14]

The same can be said for the fluidity of agency. The process of locating agency for people with diabetes is, therefore, partially dependent on space because knowing where things happen is critical to knowing how and why they happen (Warf & Arias, 2009). Re-mapping the articulations of agency in spaces of care in health care can give "a new definition of the status of the patient in society" (Foucault, 1994, p. 196), but as Foucault (1994) also states, this requires "the patient to be enveloped in a collective, homogeneous space" (p. 196). If this space is not the medical neighborhood, however, what other models might move us past the binary spaces of work and clinic? Discussions of distributed work from technical communication, the concept of *betweenity* from disability studies, and Foucault's (1984a) notion of heterotopias are useful. The common denominator of these models is that they are spaces of liminality.

Liminality, first defined by anthropologist Van Gennep (1960), has been viewed as a middle stage in rites of passage such as coming-of-age rituals and marriages. When someone moves from one social status to another, they go through a transition marked by three phases: separation, margin/limen, and reaggregation. During this middle phase, the person making the passage becomes ambiguous and this ambiguity makes the person structurally, if not physically, invisible "in terms of his culture's standard definitions and classifications" (Turner, 1974, p. 232). Here, borders and border crossings are not static nor are they one-time events. As multiple events, they do help account for the way people with diabetes shift sources of knowledge, subjectivities, and identities.

---

14. Mountford (2001) also said physical rhetorical space "is the geography of a communicative event, and, like all landscapes, may include both the cultural and material arrangement, whether intended or fortuitous, of a location" (p. 41). Her idea of rhetorical space comes out of the rhetorical situation, but Mountford also argues that rhetorical space can be a useful concept for rhetoricians, if it is applied "more narrowly" (p. 41) to physical spaces, such as rooms, confession booths, and online platforms. Applegarth's (2014) work with rhetorical archaeology also privileges space (as well as context). As she puts it, space is central to anthropology and, therefore, can offer insights to rhetorical scholars interested in "seeking spatial dimensions of rhetorical practice" (p. 19).

In technical communication, such liminal spaces have been discussed as spaces that merge work and life (Spinuzzi, Hart-Davidson, & Zachry, 2006). McNely (2014) also notes that hybrid spaces are increasing in our everyday experiences. Swartz and Kim (2009) define hybrid spaces as "meshed" locales where the symbolic and the material are hybridized and "information is not only a commodity; it is a frame on the world around us" (p. 212). Distributed work can also be seen as liminal in that it "splices together divergent work activities (separated by time, space, organizations, and objectives) and that enables the transformations of information and texts that characterize such work" (Spinuzzi, 2007, p. 265). In such spaces, texts coordinate how individuals and organizations share information, expertise, and authority (Slattery, 2007). These activities are linked to representations of symbolic analytic workers who "possess the abilities to identify, rearrange, circulate, abstract, and broker information" (Johnson-Eilola, 1996, p. 255).

In disability studies, Brueggemann reminds us that *betweenity* can be agential because being between is about potentiality (Brueggemann & Voss, n.d.). Furthermore, it is a space that is relational, rhetorical, educational, and mediated. The deaf spaces Brueggemann discusses are relational spaces between a person's various identities. They are communicative spaces in which both the dominant culture and the "other" (i.e., the deaf person) are educated and spaces that are mediated by someone (such as a person's peers) or things (such as technology). Other disability theorists see the potential of such "between" spaces as well. These scholars suggest that the hybridity and fluidity of borderlands have a performative potential (Lewiecki-Wilson & Cellio, 2011).

Finally, Foucault explains heterotopias (as well as utopias) as sites that simultaneously reflect, contest, and invert society. Heterotopias are both localized, real, and socially produced (Foucault, 1984a; Soja, 1989). They are particularly helpful in investigating questions of agency because they bring the taken-for-granted social order into question. Furthermore, they are made up of bits of space, in that they are "capable of juxtaposing in a single real place several spaces, several sites that are in themselves incompatible" (Foucault, 1984a, para. 20). Foucault outlines six principles of heterotopias. The first is their pervasive nature. The second principle is that, while a heterotopia has a precise function within a society, it can have other functions in other societies. The third principle of heterotopias is that these spaces are able to juxtapose several spaces, including sites that are incompatible. Foucault offers an example by way of explanation: "Thus it is that the theater brings onto the rectangle of the stage, one after the other, a whole series of places that are foreign to one another; thus it is that the cinema is a very odd rectangular room, at the end of which, on a two-dimensional screen, one sees the projection of a three-dimensional space" (para. 20). The fourth principle of heterotopias is that they are linked to slices in time. These slices may be long, such as the time associated with cemeteries. Or these slices of time may be fleeting, such as the amount of time associated with a festival. The fifth principle of heterotopias is that they are not public in that they cannot be accessed by everyone. The last trait of heterotopias is that they have a function in relation to all other spaces. This function may be to create a space of illusion, such as can be done through cinema, or they can create a space that is other but real.

Examples of heterotopias offered by Persson and Richards (2008) include hospital clinics, general practitioner rooms, private homes, peer support settings, and public spaces where conversations about HIV occur. The juxtaposition of the discourses in these spaces creates fissures and buckles that, much like Edbauer's (2005) topographic assessment of the rhetorical situation, give these heterotopias a three-dimensional aspect that calls up a sense of being between that challenges binaries and speaks to multiplicity. Diabetes online patient communities and face-to-face group educational appointments are these types of spaces as well. Online spaces often function as spaces of crisis. Crisis heterotopias, according to Foucault, are reserved for people in some sort of disastrous stage in their lives. Many of the members of the TuDiabetes community find their way to the site soon after a diagnosis, which is such a period of a distress.

My last two (out of 3) pregnancies were diagnosed with GD. After both pregnancies by BG levels were back to normal at my 6 weeks checkups. Then 9 months after my last pregnancy I became very irritable, agitated, and depressed (I am usually very outgoing with days packed with fun adventures with my kids). I went to the dr, they ordered some blood work- called back diagnosing me with type 2 diabetes with a blood sugars in the 500s (no wonder I felt like crap). They immediately put me on metformin, told me to eat healthy, and exercise. Trying as best I could the numbers came down slightly but not enough. I was losing weight drastically (I am 5'6" and was weighing 113, mind you 9 months after having an 11 lb baby) I lost 12 lbs in 8 weeks! After some of my own research I called and insisted on seeing an endocrinologist and asked if I could do the blood work for LADA t1. Long story short they changed my diagnosis to LADA T1. I am still struggling to keep my numbers within normal range. I have gained back some of the weight. I am currently taking troujeo (sp?) slow acting at bedtime, and glipizide before breakfast. My biggest questions are any advice for someone who is having a tough time wrapping my head around this loss of freedom.

I am raising 3 small kids all under the age of 5 and trying to balance both. I am terrified of the stories of people slipping into comas due to hyper or hypo. What happens if that occurs when I am alone with my kids and end up in the hospital? I have done research on the Internet and read some books but I continue to find conflicting information. Please help me find courage and strength to live a long healthy life to be there for my kids.

This person, like many new members of the community, is in crisis both physically, with extremely high blood glucose readings in the 500s, and psychologically by being in denial. As a member of a crisis heterotopia, she came to the space of her own free will. Face-to-face appointments, however, often bear more resemblance to heterotopias of deviation reserved for people whose behavior is somehow deviant. Foucault's examples included psychiatric hospitals and prisons. People who go to group appointments are deviant because their doctors identify them as such by their A1C percentages. The physician (Dr. Jackson) I interviewed, for example, *prescribed* group medical appointments for his patients with A1Cs greater than 7 percent.

Both heterotopias of crisis and those of deviation "presuppose a system of opening and closing that both isolates them and makes them penetrable. In general, the heterotopic site is not freely accessible like a public place. . . . To get in one must have a certain permission and make certain gestures" (Foucault, 1984a, para. 24). Certainly this is true of patient online communities. In the TuDiabetes community, such gestures include being knowledgeable about one's disease. When someone posts an initial diagnosis/request for help, responses differ in relation to the level of detail in the post. Messages written with a great deal of detail, like the following example, chain out (i.e., receive many responses).

I am new here and fairly new to Type 2. I really don't want to believe I have this crazy disease. I'm 47 and I really hate having to go through this. I'm a little heavy set lol I thought I would use that one, and I have had high blood sugar levels as far as I know for about 1 year. I am now on Metformin (maxed out) Glyburide (maxed out) and Byetta 10 MICgrams. When I started taking the byetta it helped a lot and I think my lowest reading was 170 but after about 3 months now I'm back up to 250 to 280. Maybe its because I eat wrong. Am Type 1 now?? Is oral medications and Byetta just not going to work for me? I try to change my diet somewhat but I of course struggle with that. I work 2nd shift in a plant so I get some exercise but probably not enough. A little more history I take blood pressure medicine and it has been doing great! I Play bass and sing and harmonize in a praise band at church.

(I love that.) You know they have a lot of good food at the church LOL To sum up I already gave up smoking Hooray! Don't drink anymore to speak of Hooray! But now I have to watch what I eat?? I know I can still eat good things that arent too bad for me but watching that and handling that 24 hrs a day is a bummer. What things are left in life to enjoy? Yes I know what you are thinking there is still that. I guess what I'm asking is do I need insulin? Can I eat what I want or is that now just out of the question even with medicine? Hope i get some replies. I'm a little frustrated with this whole thing. I have a feeling I am going to get an answer back that my ears won't want to hear but Im sure it will be for my own good. Give it to me straight and don't sugar coat it. hahah Am I going downhill the way I'm going?

Shorter, less informative posts such as the following are not greeted by as many responses: "i am new here and don't really know what i am supposed to do so please bare with me, i would love to chat." The fact that these more detailed posts chain out more successfully would indicate that members are more readily accepted when they express a particular value held by the group: knowledge of the disease (Arduser, 2011). By already exhibiting knowledge of the disease, the contributor is establishing her legitimacy and the right to take part in the conversation on the site.

As such, expertise is linked to a form of narrative competence, "the capacity to recognize, absorb, metabolize, interpret, and be moved by stories of illness" (Charon, 2007, p. 1265). In describing the program in narrative medicine at Columbia University Medical Center, Charon (2007) states that the goal of the program is to provide a variety of people, including doctors, nurses, social workers, psychoanalysts, and literary scholars, "rigorous training in close reading, attentive listening, reflective writing, and bearing witness to suffering" (p. 1265). People with diabetes can be seen as doing a similar thing in a more organic way. Diabetics do not need to learn to bear witness to someone else's disease but rather to their own. We can see the effects of bearing witness when a person joins the TuDiabetes community; the gesture of showing one's expertise at this early stage interpellates the individual as someone willing to share their expertise with others and, therefore, the person is accepted as a member of this community. Group appointments, which require unacceptable A1C levels for entrance, similarly use these numbers as a form of permission to enter this space. The liminal spaces I examined are, therefore, less egalitarian than the "communitas" Turner (1974, p. 45) discussed, reflecting a power differential similar to the one Jeyaraj's (2004) technical writers experience in relation to the more powerful subject matter experts and the colonized places Bhabha (1994) studied.

LIMINALITY'S RISKS TO AGENCY

As liminal spaces, online networking communities and group appointment spaces carry the risk of being non-agential as well as agential, but because agency is the result of temporary articulations, this is to be expected. One way agency is impeded in these spaces is through peer surveillance that encourages the policing of others. In a group appointment setting, for example, another person's peers will make judgments about a person's success in conducting self-management activities, and patients will classify themselves into groups that may have moralistic implications of being *good* or *bad* patients. In fact, my physician informant said that in his group, "It's obvious they have a certain accountability with colleagues that they don't always have in an office visit with me." A psychologist at one of the face-to-face group meetings I attended also said there is accountability in group meetings and appointments because patients have to report to each other.

This accountability can evoke the spoiled identity constructed for people in much of the medical text and talk about diabetes. This implication is similar to that found in the literature on the geography of AIDS in which a "discourse of blame" is constructed (Crampton & Elden, 2007). The following example from an online health article illustrates how people with diabetes use similar discourse: "He [the doctor] literally raised his voice and yelled at me like I was a child. He told me 'Yes, we could change this metformin, but you can quickly run through all the oral medications for diabetes, then you're not going to be left with any choice but insulin,'" (Metcalf, 2008). In the group appointment I went to for recruiting purposes, one woman described her eating habits in talking about her recent self-management activities, saying, "I know that's bad." She obviously attached blame to her decision to ignore the dietary advice she had received. Her high blood sugar numbers reinforced this morality, as these numbers are seen as the punishment for such transgressions. The specter of noncompliance becomes associated with being a "bad person" or "bad diabetic" (Peel et al., 2005, p. 785), and people often take on this role of disobedient child (Broom & Whittaker, 2004). In a group appointment setting, the question of who scrutinizes another's actions changes. Rather than the medical provider, the person's peers may provide surveillance. Whether purposeful or not, group educational spaces may make use of both self-surveillance and governmentality, which "incorporates both techniques or practices of the self—self-government—and the more apparent forms of external government—policing, surveillance and regulatory activities carried out by agencies of the state or other institutions for strategic purposes" (Lupton, 1995, p. 9).

Another way that agency gets obstructed is through people with diabetes turning on each other. Talking about this infighting, Jamie, one of my focus group participants, said, "Another thing that happens but should be off limits is the type 1 versus type 2 that we seem to get every so often. Sort of whose diabetes is more difficult to manage, who's more blameworthy." When I asked her to clarify what she meant by "blameworthy," Jamie answered:

Well, a few of the threads have started with somebody coming on and saying something like "I think that type 2 diabetics are responsible for having brought this disease on themselves and I don't like to be lumped in with type 2 diabetes. I think it's really unfortunate that the media lumps us all in together because type 2 cause their own disease." And there are some threads that have hundreds and hundreds of posts that started off with something like that. And it's just utterly unhelpful to anybody, I think, to have that discussion over and over. You get the entire gamut of responses to people who agree with the original poster to people who think that that's total B. S. to people who feel guilty themselves, you know, type 2 diabetics who say, "you know, I didn't eat very well you know, maybe I am responsible for having brought this on myself." Then eventually I guess that people get bored with the thread and it tends to go away. But then it'll come back later.

The following reaction to an insulting post took place on a TuDiabetes' member's blog:

Similarly, I'm tired of the stereotyping of type 2 diabetics that goes on on this site, because the intention is the same: to affix blame, and to make some kind of moral argument that type 2 diabetics brought on their disease through poor choices (calling type 2 a "lifestyle disease") whereas type 1 diabetics are morally pristine [. . .].

A similar post on a discussion forum receives a sarcastic congratulatory reply:

I was diagnosed a little over 3 months ago, and I cannot tell you how annoying I think it is when people at work, say "oh look what I found online to prevent diabetes, Martin you should take a look." I CANT STAND IT!! Believe me, I am well aware that these people are my supporters and are only trying to help, but I feel like Type 1 diabetics are so much different than Type 2. First off, Type 1 diabetics can do absolutely NOTHING to cause this, so right off the bat we are 100% helpless. Not to dis Type 2 diabetics, but I feel like they brought the diabetes upon themselves. Had there been ANYTHING I could

have done to cause my Type 1, believe me, I would take complete responsibility. I guess it is probably a lack of information for the average person to
know the difference between Type 1 and Type 2, but I find it very annoying
when a person categorizes me with a Type 2. Another reason it bothers me
is because not only did they bring it on themselves, but they don't have to
do injections, or monitor their sugar NEARLY as frequently as we Type 1's.

The post received 240 responses, including the following one: "Congratula-
tions on being a type 1. hope you enjoy the lack of guilt." As this comment
indicates, unlike the victim role occupied by type 1 diabetes in public discourse, the public discourse surrounding type 2 in the community of people
with diabetes is much more similar to the medical discourse about diabetics
generally. Type 2, seen as an "earned" disease, often focuses on issues of willpower and blame. These divisions or dis-articulations magnify my argument
that people with diabetes are not a singular patient set, as they are represented
to be in much of the medical research and literature. People with diabetes, it
appears, do not always feel a sense of community but they are bound together
as one as Linton (1998) so vividly describes in talking about people with disabilities: "We may drool, hear voices, speak in staccato syllables, wear cath-
eters to collect our urine, or live with a compromised immune system. We are
all bound together, not by this list of our collective symptoms but by the social
and political circumstances that have forged us as a group" (p. 4).

OVERLAPPING DISCOURSE AND LIMINAL AGENCY

In spite of the articulations of disease, blame, and victimhood, the nature of
liminal spaces as "ambiguous spatiality" (Hetherington, 1997, p. 42) defies easy
classifications and as such has a transformative power. They are particularly
helpful in investigating questions of agency because they bring the taken-for-
granted social order into question. Overlapping spaces allow inhabitants to
subvert the narratives of established power and dominant cultures (Bhabha,
1994) and enhance knowledge exchange by allowing participants to question, challenge, reinterpret, and renegotiate identity. Border crossings within
these spaces occur through the juxtaposition of the competing discourses of
lived experience and clinical medical knowledge of both people with diabetes
and medical professionals. As these competing discourses vibrate against one
another, as they do in group and online settings, diabetics renegotiate articulations much like folk dancers change partners to reposition themselves.

When the spaces of the home and clinic overlap, resources exist for patients to enact rhetorical agency by providing alternative discourses to draw from: the discourse of the medical providers they interact with and the discourse of lived experience provided by other patients. Collaborative spaces allow for the entry of discourse that competes with a biomedical discourse established on clinical research and vetted by doctors. Responses from my provider participants about patient interaction verify the existence of this discourse in their experiences with group appointments. Daisy, the CDE, for example, said,

> But anyway, this—learning in a group—is more secure for a lot of people. They feel we-are-in-this-together type of thing. And I don't have to say anything if I don't want to. I don't have to show my ignorance if that's what I am afraid of. I don't have to be embarrassed to reveal something if I have heard other people talk about what they did, and nobody got mad or laughed at them. So it gives them confidence, I think, to be in a group. Since I've done a lot of group things, more so in the last few years, I learn something almost every class because if you really listen to people, they are revealing something about themselves and how they deal with things. If you're really listening, you'll hear something usable that might help somebody else. If they have solved a problem some way or another, there may be another person that could use that idea too.

As Daisy suggests, hearing about the similar experience of another person with diabetes is powerful in these settings. This similar experience is very individual—so much so that people in the online TuDiabetes community are particular about who they received advice from, an idea I explore more in depth in chapter 4. Many of my focus group participants talked about going to another member's profile to check that person's A1C, making sure it was at an acceptable level before believing a solution the person offered for a problem on the discussion forums. Sara, one community member and focus group participant, went so far as to check to see if the other member had the same form of diabetes as she did and used the same technology for treatment before being willing to listen to that person's advice.

> SARA: I've gone back and checked the person's profile, checking what their last A1C is. I will have to admit to being biased and looking specifically to seeing if they are type 1, and if they're on the pump or daily injections. And to check to see what some of their other responses to other questions have been.

Along with bringing in new authoritative voices that have traditionally been marginalized, assumptions about power and authority can be challenged and the counter narratives that emerge are an expression of rhetorical agency. Drawing on the competing discourse of lived experience, for instance, complicates the biomedical definition of control, as is evident in the responses from my focus group when asked about defining control:

GRACE: I guess for me it's still being alive and not having any really bad complications. I know of some diabetics 50 years going and they can barely see or move, and that scares the heck out of me because I'm nearing the 50 years [of living with diabetes]. But they're still alive and they still have a good sense of humor about them. I mean, that's the way I cope with my problems. I just have to joke about it. Maybe that's the way all of you are with diabetes.

MARY: From a different perspective, for me being in control means having an A1C that is as close to 6 as possible and being on no meds. But that's type 2.

DAVID: I guess I can see two sides of it. Not that I like to use the scare tactics of "you're going to lose a leg and you're going to lose your eye sight," but I really value my legs and my eye sight, so I think keeping that in check as a typical modality of not taking care of my disease is pretty motivating. But I also look at the fact that I enjoy running. I enjoy cycling. I enjoy being able to eat pretty much any food I want, you know, in the proper portions. But I like being able to live my life the way I want to live it, so I guess the best way I can do that is to maintain proper control and really understand the disease and stay on top of the disease so I can continue doing the things that I like to do.

This exchange shows that although the biomedical concept of control (being within or below a numerical target) is prevalent in the discussions of people with diabetes in these spaces, there is room to discuss control in a very different way. Although Mary, the type 2 participant, ties her definition of control to her A1C value, all of the interviewees with type 1 in this discussion related control to various aspects of their lives rather than a numeric value. Control is taken out of the context of their disease and applied to their entire life. The competing discourse of people's lived experience allows us to not only see the person with diabetes, which we cannot do in the medical neighborhood as currently presented, but also see a more complicated version of a person with diabetes.

WRITING AND LIMINAL AGENCY

Liminal spaces also open up possibilities for people with diabetes to be more than recorders of their body's information. These activities give people with diabetes a form of agency that historically has been seen as emerging from the process of writing and the assumption that language is power.[15] In liminal spaces, people with diabetes are able to enact agency through writing in ways unavailable to them in other spaces. However, the relationship of interest in these spaces is that of the writer and the audience rather than the writer and the text. It is the process of this transformation that opens the space for a concept of agency to exist that is similar to the one Miller (2007) argued for in her work with composition instructors. In this study, Miller concluded that "agency can be understood as the kinetic energy of performance that is generated through a process of mutual attribution between rhetor and audience" (p. 137).

Norm, at age 83 and living with diabetes since 1968, is writing a memoir of which he said, "I just kind of do something to help others deal with this." Online people write blogs. One member of a focus group, introducing herself as a "Jill of all trades," talked about her blogging activities on diabetes. Another told us that her doctor had been encouraging her to share her story and knowledge through blog writing. Blog writing, as a genre, has shifted from a form of diary writing or journaling to a writing form in which there is an expectation for interaction between a writer and the readers.[16] In the case of my focus group participants, the goal of this interaction is to share information and help other people with diabetes. As Grace said when telling the focus group about her work as a blogger, "I've had diabetes pretty well all my life. And actually diabetes has paid off for me now. I work in this area, so it's great. I can help people out." Mary, who had been diagnosed in 2008, was undertaking a similar project with the encouragement of her physician:

---

15. Much of the scholarship on workplace studies in technical communication has focused on writing (see Henry, 2000; Spilka, 1993; Duin and Hansen, 1996; as well as several of the books in the Association of Teachers of Technical Writing (ATTW) Contemporary Studies in Communication series). This scholarship is largely informed by the 1993 text of Slack et al. in which they examine the relationship between technical communicators and the notion of authorship. They argue that to grant authorship to a discourse is to privilege and valorize it. Technical communication has not been viewed as an authored discourse and, therefore, technical communicators have not been viewed as authors or agents but as transmitters or translators of information.

16. See Miller and Shepherd (2004) and (2009).

He said, you know, "You need to share your story, you have all this knowl-edge of how you did this. You got off the meds and you need to get online and sort of let people know that and pass that on." So that's why I sort of said, "Okay." I'm not the most gregarious person in the world so, you know, I said, "Let's try it online."

Many members of online patient communities also author discourse by regularly participating in discussion forums. One member of a focus group commented:

I tend to [respond to a post], like if someone's newly diagnosed it depends on the question and if I feel like I can answer it best because there's some people on TuDiabetes they should be doctors, they're so well educated in diabetes. But I'll respond and I'll either point them in another direction in TuDiabetes and I guess just wish them good luck.

As Johndan Johnson-Eilola (1996) noted, symbolic analysts in the contempo-rary information economy must create, manage, and distribute digital media as well as textual documents. In the case of people with diabetes, this work is also apparent in shared spaces. People make videos for online patient commu-nity sites and YouTube. Vlogger DiabeticDanica, for example, regularly shares tutorials for using technologies such as insulin pumps on YouTube for other people with type 1 diabetes. Danica, who has been diabetic for 15 years, has over 10,000 followers on YouTube as well as an active presence on Facebook, Instagram, and Twitter.

In face-to-face spaces that include a medical professional, people with diabetes also enact agency through writing. In the handout with the ladder diagram I mentioned in the previous chapter, for instance, patients write their goals down, not the medical provider. Although this writing is often seen as agential by medical authorities because it is inventive and encourages owner-ship of goals, this type of writing is actually an act of compliance. In describing the end of one of her group sessions, a pharmacist who was interviewed said,

So then we go through the material of the class. Then at the end I will go around and take blood pressures one by one and weights. You know, blood pressure, weight, blood pressure, weight, blood pressure, weight. But before I do blood pressures and weights I say, "Now you need to write a goal for the next time."

This direction in itself might be seen as being similar to a prompt used in any writing class, a way to help students with rhetorical invention. However, the pharmacist said that when she starts her class for the next session she will say, "You set a goal last week of . . . you know . . . eating breakfast at least every day. Did you meet that goal?" Or, "You said you're gonna exercise twice a week for 30 minutes. Did you meet that goal?" So we discuss that at the beginning of class." This statement puts less focus on making meaning than on complying with goals they set. Writing as such becomes an act of accountability or compliance rather than an act of invention. However, in both online and face-to-face spaces, people with diabetes do draw on oral storytelling, an interactive and relational activity that requires a call and response that creates mutual or collaborative invention. In a discussion thread about advice on a particular kind of insulin pump (the OmniPod), for example, a community member says,

> Hi George, well I know for myself absorption is different depending on where I put the pod. works well for me on the buttocks, thighs arms, and on the girls. lol I know some ppl also use it by there love handles. my best site is on the girls, then back of arms, back and then thighs. . . .

These two people go back and forth:

> ORIGINAL POSTER: Thanks for the response Harry. After a slight high after breakfast today is going well. I totally agree about the freedom, it's a bit of a weird feeling having it stuck to my arm but I can live with that one!
> RESPONDER: do you drink coffee in the morning? I notice that if I have more then a cup of coffee 2 or more, that I put in 2 units to compensate and my sugars stay stable.

Other people join the conversation, then the original two reappear:

> RESPONDER: The pods can only be used maximum 3 days. Dex will only guarantee for a week but ppl have had them working for 3 weeks or more.
> ORIGINAL POSTER: Thanks you to all who have responded to my question and given me some helpful guidance. I am liking the OmniPod and still learning how to get the best from it, and thank you for all the tips! I'm having better days since changing from that original problem site. I have to say on a good day the OmniPod is great and so much better than my old tube pump!

In online patient communities, people will post prompts such as "Re-using lancets—some thoughts." This prompt starts a dialogue with other members of the community who contribute to the discussion about whether or not they reuse the device to draw blood from a fingertip to test their blood sugar levels on a home glucose (blood sugar) meter. As such, the relationship that is important here is that between the person posting and the responding audience. The pharmacists I interviewed describe a similar call and response pattern in their group appointments. In describing the interaction between patients in a shared medical appointment, a pharmacist told me,

> It seems like there's more communication back and forth. There's more inter-action when there's two people [patients]. When there's one person that one person may not ask as much or respond as deeply. They kind of play off each other: One will ask a question another will ask a related question, and they'll kind of go from there.

Such call and response patterns are patterns of interaction between a speaker and listener in which all *calls* are accompanied by an expression (*response*) from the listener. In music this pattern is defined as a musical phrase in which the first part (which is often a solo part) is answered by a second part, which is often an ensemble part. Here, the call and response may be the back and forth that goes on in a discussion thread online. Rather than agency being defined by the relationship between a writer and her text or a speaker and a listening audience, these interactions can be agential by virtue of the articulations between the people *in the room*, whether that is a physical or virtual meeting place.

The concepts of heterotopias, *betweenity*, and liminality are important in spaces in which articulations form because, as Hall (1986) states, articulations are not rigid and eternal. As such, agency is not a given but must be negotiated by formulating agential connections between different forms of knowledge, subjectivities, and identities. As this chapter has shown, two ways of doing this are through negotiating multiple overlapping discourses and engaging in writing as a relational activity. Both of these performances of agency in liminal spaces can inform ways patients and medical providers interact in more stable spaces and encourage new definitions of patient agency.

CHAPTER 3

Rhetorical Plasticity

Negotiating Types of Knowledge

I often say to people, "I wish people had a little spot on their forehead that would turn red when their blood sugar went over 140." So far that hasn't happened. . . . So knowing what your blood sugar is, thinking about what your blood sugar may have been earlier: That's why testing is so important. It's pure information.

—Daisy, CDE

IF MUCH of the work of diabetes is of a symbolic-analytic nature, we need to ask what knowledge looks like for these workers and how this knowledge is agential. To become expert, people with diabetes do need to acquire specialized knowledge, but the way this acquisition is represented by medical professionals and the texts they create and the way people with diabetes actually acquire knowledge and make meaning are vastly at odds. Medical texts and talk emphasize a transmission model of knowledge production (Slack et al., 1993), a model tied to the idea of messages being transported.[1] This metaphor is clearly apparent in the language medical professionals use (think back to Daisy and the car) and tied to a motif of journeys. This epistemology encourages a view of agency as a possession that can be transferred from one individual to another through an exchange of knowledge and skills. Once a patient has received the necessary knowledge from the medical expert, the patient is expert and has agency—the capacity to act in a way that will result in controlled blood sugar levels in diabetes care. Within such a worldview, patients progress from a stance of learning *about* to learning *how*. The fol-

---

1. Such a view was largely shaped by Shannon and Weaver's (1948) linear model of communication in which a sender transmits meaning to a receiver. The message is sent over a channel to the receiver who decodes it in order to get meaning from the message. If communication was successful, the receiver decodes exactly the same message that the sender intended to send.

lowing excerpt is an example of how the dietitian I interviewed, Susan, used the phrases *learn about* and *learn how* in a conversation about knowledge acquisition.

> SUSAN: Well, in the first hour of the class we give them a meal-planning guide from the Diabetic Association [ADA] that they need to plan themselves while I'm sitting there. You know, they sit there, they *learn all about* [emphasis added] the carbohydrates and *learn about* [emphasis added] how many they're supposed to have per day and per meal. And then they have to do it themselves. So I really encourage people to, it's kind of like you give a man a fish he'll have a meal but if you teach him how to fish he'll eat forever. I really want them to *learn how* [emphasis added] to plan their own meals because it's not like I'm going to be shadowing them at home. But for a lot of people, they really want to be told what they're supposed to eat at every meal and every snack. And while that's nice and it makes me feel good, I also find it kind of sad that they don't take the initiative themselves to find out, "Okay, well this has so many grams of carbohydrate, so I can either have this or I can have this." So I kind of wish they were more empowered but some of them just either don't want to do it or just kind of make so many excuses not to.

The process for this acquisition is presented as a linear one. First, a person has to acquire the specialized knowledge (episteme), then the skill (techne) can be practiced. This linearity is obvious on organizational websites, such as those of the American Diabetes Association and the National Diabetes Education Program (NDEP). The American Diabetes Association's (ADA) Blood Glucose Control web page, for example, gives specific instructions for checking blood sugar at home with a blood glucose meter. These instructions take a step approach by providing a procedure or accomplishing a physical or mental task.

How do I check?

1. After washing your hands, insert a test strip into your meter.
2. Use your lancing device on the side of your fingertip to get a drop of blood.
3. Gently squeeze or massage your finger until a drop of blood forms. (Required sample sizes vary by meter.)

4. Touch and hold the edge of the test strip to the drop of blood, and wait for the result.
5. Your blood glucose level will appear on the meter's display.[2]

An examination of a document produced by the NDEP further exemplifies just how people with diabetes are represented as technicians (people who use information rather than produce knowledge) who first acquire information and then use practical knowledge to engage in practical tasks. The NDEP's main web page for people with diabetes is arranged as a series of steps:

- Step 1: Learn About Diabetes
- Step 2: Know Your Diabetes ABCs
- Step 3: Manage Your Diabetes
- Step 4: Get Routine Care to Avoid Problems

This text focuses on first defining terms and the disease before moving on to explaining how to care for it. In Step 1, the patient is introduced to the disease with definitions of the most prevalent types: type 1, type 2, and gestational diabetes. Step 1 then moves to a call to action:

Diabetes is serious.

You may have heard people say they have "a touch of diabetes" or "your sugar is a little high." These words suggest that diabetes is not a serious disease. That is not correct. Diabetes is serious, but you can learn to manage it! All people with diabetes need to make healthy food choices, stay at a healthy weight, and be physically active every day.

Following this call is a brief discussion of some of the major complications that can be a result of the disease. Step 2 reinforces the position of the patient as a student or apprentice with its title:

Step 2: Know Your Diabetes ABCs. (A1C, Blood Pressure, and Cholesterol)
Talk to your health care team about how to manage your A1C (blood glucose or sugar), **B**lood pressure, and **C**holesterol. This will help lower your chances of having a heart attack, a stroke, or other diabetes problems. Here's what the ABCs of diabetes stand for:

---

2. Copyright © 2013–2015 American Diabetes Association. From www.diabetes.org. Reprinted with permission from the American Diabetes Association.

A for the A1C test.
The A1C Test shows you what your blood glucose has been over the last three months. The A1C goal for many people is below 7. High blood glucose levels can harm your heart and blood vessels, kidneys, feet, and eyes.

B for Blood pressure.
The blood pressure goal for most people with diabetes is below 140/90. It may be different for you. Ask what your goal should be.

High blood pressure makes your heart work too hard. It can cause heart attack, stroke, and kidney disease.

C for Cholesterol.
Ask what your cholesterol numbers should be.

LDL or "bad" cholesterol can build up and clog your blood vessels. It can cause a heart attack or a stroke. HDL or "good" cholesterol helps remove cholesterol from your blood vessels.

The language in this step brings to mind an image of an elementary school child, a time when people are learning the alphabet. The information included on the page is brief and definitional as in Step 1. In Step 3, reproduced in part here, the patient has learned the material and now must practice. In this step, the reader is given 12 things he can do as part of a self-care plan to manage the disease.

Many people avoid the long-term problems of diabetes by taking good care of themselves. Work with your health care team to reach your ABC goals (A1C, Blood Pressure, Cholesterol): Use this self-care plan.

- Use your diabetes meal plan. If you do not have one, ask your health care team about one.
- Make healthy food choices such as fruits and vegetables, fish, lean meats, chicken or turkey without the skin, dry peas or beans, whole grains, and low-fat or skim milk and cheese.
- Keep fish and lean meat and poultry portion to about 3 ounces (or the size of a deck of cards). Bake, broil, or grill it.
- Eat foods that have less fat and salt.

TABLE 4. Health Provider's Perceived Role in Step 3

HEALTH PROVIDER AS RESOURCE	HEALTH PROVIDER AS INTERPRETER
❑ Use your diabetes meal plan. If you do not have one, ask your health care team about one.	❑ Take medicines even when you feel good. Ask your doctor if you need aspirin to prevent a heart attack or stroke. Tell your doctor if you cannot afford your medicines or if you have any side effects.
❑ Stay at a healthy weight by using your meal plan and moving more.	❑ Check your feet every day for cuts, blisters, red spots, and swelling. Call your health care team right away about any sores that do not go away.
❑ Ask for help if you feel down. A mental health counselor, support group, member of the clergy, friend, or family member who will listen to your concerns may help you feel better.	❑ Check your blood glucose (blood sugar). You may want to test it one or more times a day. Use the card at the back of this booklet to keep a record of your blood glucose numbers. Be sure to take this record to your doctor visits.
❑ Stop smoking. Ask for help to quit.	❑ Check your blood pressure if your doctor advises.
	❑ Report any changes in your eyesight to your doctor.

These and the other 11 items list things patients should do. As such, the self-care plan would seem to empower patients, foregrounding their actions with the focus on the verbs in these bullets. The rest of the bulleted text, however, is written in language that foregrounds doctors rather than patients. In the first bullet, for example, the text says that if you do not have a meal plan, you should "ask your health care team about one." The health care team's role in this language is presented as either a resource or an interpreter (table 4). When positioned as a resource, the person with diabetes has more agency. When positioned an interpreter, the health care provider has more agency.

Interestingly, the text that seems the most empowering, the two bulleted lists separated by text at the bottom of the page, places the patient closest to the same level as physician. The lead-in for this bulleted list states: "Actions you could take." These actions are as follows:

- Talk with your health care team about your blood glucose targets. Ask how and when to test your blood glucose and how to use the results to manage your diabetes.
- Discuss how your self-care plan is working for you each time you visit your health care team.

Leading with the word "could" suggests the reader has a choice, which would be empowering, but by separating this text with space from the other text, this message is de-emphasized. Step 4, the final step, maintains a bullet-list format but shifts away from the starting verb construction.

See your health care team at least twice a year to find and treat any problems early. Ask what steps you can take to reach your goals.

If you have diabetes, at each visit be sure you have a:
- blood pressure check
- foot check
- weight check
- review of your self-care plan shown in Step 3

If you have diabetes, two times each year get:
- A1C test—it may be checked more often if it is over 7

If you have diabetes, once each year be sure you have a:
- cholesterol test
- triglyceride (try-GLISS-er-ide) test—a type of blood fat
- complete foot exam
- dental exam to check teeth and gums—tell your dentist you have diabetes
- dilated eye exam to check for eye problems
- flu shot
- urine and a blood test to check for kidney problems

By starting with an opening clause and burying the verb related to patient action in the sentence, the provider is once again the focus of the story and the providers' role is emphasized, which emphasizes epistemic knowledge gained from a provider. Like the managed care educational materials that Stone (1997) analyzed, the four steps are designed to empower patients by encouraging them to become more involved in their own care. However, the materials that Stone examined and this example also illustrate that the established language conventions of medical discourse are at work in these texts and this discourse restrains patient agency as defined in this book. The NDEP text still reflects the standard imbalance of power in the doctor/patient relationship and continues to use the conceptual framework of the medical community and the language of the compliance paradigm.

While the NDEP text emphasizes episteme and the ADA text emphasizes techne, both mask the performer (the patient). As such, these texts assume a mechanical reality with facts being self-evident and existing out there in the real world or as something we simply need to capture and put to use. Instruction sets, as the examples from the ADA and the NDEP websites indicate, are often presented as a series of steps and center on events that are contingent on each other and ordered chronologically. They also emphasize procedure over understanding (Selber, 2010). Procedural discourse, like that used to explain how to test blood sugar, relegates such skills to the realm of operationalism and ignores the impact of human judgment on such acts. Therefore, much like the instructional documentation Sauer (2003) discussed, these kinds of step instructions are rhetorically incomplete. As Sauer (2003) explains: "Despite the apparent certainty of the numbers, rational, rule-based procedures, this seemingly ordered list of procedures provides insufficient information for making judgments about risk in an uncertain environment" (p. 201). Unlike the instructional text Sauer looks at from the U.S. Department of Labor's *Roof and Rib Control Manual,* the documentation created for people with diabetes does not call on the reader to use his or her own lived experience to draw conclusions. Instead, it refers the reader back to the health care team. Step 4 specifically states, "See your health care team at least twice a year to find and treat any problems early."

RE-ARTICULATING EPISTEMIC KNOWLEDGE AND INTERPRETATION

The prioritization of epistemic knowledge, as well as the certainty of numbers discussed in chapter 1, is no surprise and is evident in a variety of ways. One example of this precedence is evident in our university structures in the United States. Curricula emphasize theoretical knowledge as students become more and more specialized when earning higher degrees. As undergraduates, students take a broad range of classes. When they enter advanced degree programs they begin to concentrate more closely on theoretical concepts related to those specializations. Evidence-based medicine puts a similar primacy on epistemic knowledge. An evidence-based paradigm of medicine works under the assumption that "when possible, clinicians use information derived from systematic, reproducible, and unbiased studies to increase their confidence in the true prognosis, efficacy or therapy, and usefulness of diagnostic tests. Clinical guidelines are necessary to bring this information to those places where clinical knowledge is applied: Doctors' offices and clinical wards" (Timmermans & Berg, 2003, p. 88).

The American Diabetes Association's *Standards of Medical Care* provides a clear example of this assumption. The standards evolved from several research studies, including the *Diabetes Control and Complications Trial* (DCCT) and the *United Kingdom Prospective Diabetes Study* (UKPDS). They include recommendations for screening, diagnosis, and treatment of diabetes (figure 3) with a grading system to "clarify and codify the evidence that forms the basis for the recommendations" (ADA, 2016, p. S2). The system not only provides the criteria used in forming the guidelines and recommendations in the standard of care, but also grades or prioritizes the evidence used.[3] The grading system prioritizes pure science (randomized control trials with adequate statistical power) over applied science (clinical experience), the technical skills people with diabetes use in their day-to-day self-management practice.

Such classification systems generate hierarchies, and these hierarchies give power to disciplines that are closest to research (basic science) and the making of theoretical knowledge or episteme. Here, the researchers who carried out the *Diabetes Control and Complications Trial* and the *United Kingdom Prospective Diabetes Study* are at the top of the hierarchy as scientific knowledge because the research projects are based on clinical trials. Expert consensus or clinical experience is given less credibility and importance than well-controlled, generalizable, randomized controlled trials, which are quantitative, comparative, controlled experiments. The practicing providers—like the physician, the certified diabetes educator, the pharmacists, and the dietitian I interviewed for this study—fall into the middle of the hierarchy as applied scientists. They carry out actions informed by the knowledge someone else creates. Although they are not knowledge producers, they use and share knowledge in their interactions with patients. Patients are located at the bottom of this hierarchy, working in the day-to-day world of diabetes. These technicians (i.e., patients) could be seen as carrying out the manual work determined by the standards of care and individual treatment plans rather than producing knowledge, the task of the top tier of the hierarchy.

People with diabetes do value specialized knowledge in their day-to-day work with the disease. Several of my study participants referred to the books *Think Like a Pancreas* and *Diabetes for Dummies*. They also talked about the dLife and American Diabetes Association websites. They understood that they

---

3. It is interesting to note the contrast between the A-B-C grade construction of the first three categories, which mimic the grading systems we are used to seeing in educational settings, and the last category of "E." Unlike D or F, E does not have the educational connotations of a failing grade.

Table 1—ADA evidence-grading system for "Standards of Medical Care in Diabetes"	
Level of evidence	Description
A	Clear evidence from well-conducted, generalizable randomized controlled trials that are adequately powered, including • Evidence from a well-conducted multicenter trial • Evidence from a meta-analysis that incorporated quality ratings in the analysis Compelling nonexperimental evidence, i.e., "all or none" rule developed by the Centre for Evidence-Based Medicine at the University of Oxford Supportive evidence from well-conducted randomized controlled trials that are adequately powered, including • Evidence from a well-conducted trial at one or more institutions • Evidence from a meta-analysis that incorporated quality ratings in the analysis
B	Supportive evidence from well-conducted cohort studies • Evidence from a well-conducted prospective cohort study or registry • Evidence from a well-conducted meta-analysis of cohort studies Supportive evidence from a well-conducted case-control study
C	Supportive evidence from poorly controlled or uncontrolled studies • Evidence from randomized clinical trials with one or more major or three or more minor methodological flaws that could invalidate the results • Evidence from observational studies with high potential for bias (such as case series with comparison with historical controls) • Evidence from case series or case reports Conflicting evidence with the weight of evidence supporting the recommendation
E	Expert consensus or clinical experience

FIGURE 3. The American Diabetes Association's grading system for diabetes clinical practice. Copyright © 2016 American Diabetes Association. From *Diabetes Care*, 39 (Suppl. 1), S1–S2. Reprinted with permission from the American Diabetes Association.

needed to glean new and specialized knowledge from expert sources to educate themselves about the disease. At the same time, they saw this process as more than the transfer of knowledge. Nikki, for example, said,

Once I have knowledge, knowledge is power for me. That is what empowerment is to me. If I don't know what diabetes is, if I don't know what the dynamic between the human body and the food that we put in the human body is, if I don't know what exercise or insulin, you know, will do to my body, or medications or what have you, or what other potential medications may affect my numbers, if I don't invest time in seeking out knowledge, then I don't have any power to control it. I am at the mercy of whatever winds may come my way. And I think that we can work with them [doctors] as far as growing to learn about this disease together, but we have to be both active, actively invested people in our management of our disease.

Nikki echoes Foucault's (1980) argument that power and knowledge are linked. For her, knowledge allows her to exercise power rather than possess it. Nikki expresses this by saying that knowledge lets her "work with doctors" rather than receive treatment from doctors. This idea of working with doctors has been prevalent in documents created for use in diabetic-related contexts since at least the 1990s. Stone (1997) gives an example from Eli Lilly in her study of texts in diabetes settings:

> How you feel with diabetes is really up to you. By taking charge of your diabetes—following your health care team's instructions, keeping close track of your blood sugars, and learning all you can about your disease—you can feel better and enjoy a lower risk of complications. That's why we've created this workbook. In it, you'll find an overview of diabetes and information on ways to control it. . . . But don't forget: to best and most safely manage your diabetes, there's no substitute for the care of your health care team. So work with them. Learn all you can. You'll be on your way to a happier, healthier, and more independent life with diabetes. (as quoted in Stone, 1997, p. 207)

In such texts the patient at once "takes charge" but also "follows orders." More current texts, such as an advertisement in a popular consumer magazine for the long-acting insulin Toujeo®, echo this tension. The ad tells prospective buyers to "start a conversation with your doctor" in order to get a new prescription for this medication. And yet, the consumer is also warned not to make any changes to the amounts of Toujeo® she is injecting "without talking to your doctor." Whether taking charge or starting a conversation, the problematic relationship between agency and compliance continues to exist in medical documents. Nikki's use of the adage "work with your doctors" takes up such language, but here the doctor learns and grows with the patient. This would indicate that Nikki has more knowledge, or at least a different kind of knowledge, that the doctor can benefit from.

Another way people with diabetes reverse the "trickle down effect" of traditional notions of gaining knowledge is through their reliance on information provided by other people with diabetes. Tom, who we first met at the beginning of the book, said,

> I was recommended to a blog—buyer beware, take this with a grain of salt— *Diabetes Daily* was one of the first ones I signed up on. I only posted one

or two, but I enjoyed reading the practical things people could offer, as far as what insulin pumps they were successful with, what CGM devices they were successful with. Even how to do some of the corrections. What food had a higher glycemic index and raised your blood sugar higher, versus things that had done better. I found that educational as far as the practical aspects for disease management. The blogs were what helped me with the more practical.

According to Tom's excerpt, he not only turns to the community for information, but he engages in a process of evaluating this information. Paige echoes this activity of evaluation, but in her case, she evaluates information supplied by medical authorities. In a response to a question about where my focus group participants look for information, Paige said,

For me, I think it was just reading a lot of information on different websites, including Blood Sugar 101 and the American Association for Clinical Endocrinologists. I found it to be such a huge contrast that the American Diabetes Association tells folks to stay below 180 versus endocrinologists telling patients that they need to stay below 140 when they can, so with all the data and information that I have read documenting that most complications start taking place once patients start routinely and regularly staying at a number of 140 and higher, I tried to stay in my own personal goals below 140 and my current A1C is also below 6 percent, at 5.5 percent right now.

Paige sees knowledge to be an act of interpretation and individual judgment. She does not see knowledge as simply information to be acted upon, as the chapter's opening quotation from Daisy would suggest, however. When she found that the guidance from the American Association for Clinical Endocrinologists and the American Diabetes Association differed, she interpreted the certainty that was expressed as numeric values and applied it to her own situation. In the process of acquiring, understanding, and interpreting, people with diabetes engage in meaning making in ways the medical model of patient agency does not capture in texts based on numeric certainties that preclude any interpretation on the patient's part. If we examine the insulin sliding scale, for example, we find an exercise in pure arithmetic.[4] But people with diabetes, finding themselves in an environment in which quick decisions need to be

---

4. An example of a sliding scale can be found at www.fpnotebook.com/endo/pharm/InslnSldngScl.htm.

made, must act as symbolic analysts who, like engineers, scientists, and other "mind workers," engage in *processing* information and symbols for a living.

TECHNE AND BODILY KNOWLEDGE

In making meaning, people with diabetes do more than just rely on epistemic knowledge that is transferred unfiltered by medical specialists. Nikki does this by developing an understanding of how her body "does" diabetes. Liz seeks advice from other diabetics by reading their blogs. Paige not only reads but also compares and interprets medical guidelines to create her own goals based on her understanding of these guidelines. Along with this more robust form of epistemic knowledge, people with diabetes routinely draw on other types of knowledge. These other types are techne, which I tie to skill with technology, and bodily knowledge, which I liken to Beverly Sauer's (2003) concept of pit sense. Prior to 400 BC, techne was referred to as a craft or ability to do something and as a set of rules or theories, but discussions of the contrasts or similarities between episteme and techne have been long-standing.[5] In rhetorical studies, the contemporary links and differences between episteme, most often translated as theoretical knowledge, and techne, typically translated as craft or art, can be traced back to Aristotle and the distinctions he made in Book VI of *The Nicomachean Ethics*. In the text, Aristotle relates episteme to the scientific part (*epistemonikon*) of the rational soul that deals with certainties. The calculating/reasoning part (*logistikon*), characterized as techne, deals with things that change. Such distinctions have created a bifurcation in knowledge that continues in Western culture, with episteme more tied to a theoretical kind of knowledge that is deliberate and repeatable (scientific), as we see in the *Standards of Medical Care* for diabetes.

The distinction remains alive in the separation of creation from production as well, one which de Certeau (1984) illustrates in an example of the response of Fiat's (the car company's) leadership to the workers' attempts to talk to the leadership about their ideas about change for the organization. The workers' input was ignored because, after all, creation is the job of management. Workers just produce. Winsor's (2003) study of work that goes on in an engineering center also provides an example of the division between knowledge producing and product producing, a divide embodied in the notions

---

5. Techne has also been described as a "determinate subject matter . . . which is clearly delineated by a set of rules." (Roochnik, 1996, p. 70). Plato's use of and distinction between episteme and techne was such that Roochnik (1996) claimed that even late into Plato's career he used the terms as "virtual synonyms" (p. 277).

of white-collar and blue-collar jobs. Blue-collar workers are associated with manual labor jobs, hourly wages, and factory environments. White-collar jobs are associated with professional fields and service sector jobs, annual salaries, and offices. In Winsor's (2003) study, the engineers, the white-collar workers, are seen as producing knowledge and the technicians as the blue-collar workers carrying out the manual work task: The technicians, in other words, were interchangeable tools that were set to work by the work orders.

At times in my participant interview texts, diabetics prioritize such techne. The next excerpt gives techne priority, as evidenced by the phrase *learn how.*

> CONNIE: I had to re-educate myself as to how to carb count. I was doing it before and somehow I attained a A1C of 7 percent. I don't know how I did that. And, again, we didn't have all the testing supplies that we have now, but I had to *learn how* [emphasis added] to carb count.

Interestingly, this excerpt is from someone with type 1 diabetes, and the previous excerpt (Nikki) that focused more on knowledge/information was from someone with type 2. This distinction may be related to the onset of the disease and the fact that type 1 diabetics are more likely to use more technology than type 2 diabetics. But now, even people with type 2 diabetes sometimes use insulin pumps, or at least insulin syringes, and both type 1 and type 2 require the daily technology of the blood glucose meter. This focus on techne, therefore, comes as no surprise since people with diabetes have to have the technical skills to insert a test strip into a blood glucose meter, swab a finger with alcohol, stick it with a lancet, and squeeze a drop of blood onto the test strip. The way my participants with diabetes apply techne, unlike the way medical professionals talk about this type of knowledge, however, involves interpretation as well as action. They are required to make decisions about what to do with information, the blood sugar reading. Let's say a person tests their blood sugar and it is 180 mg/dL—it is higher than it should be. The person must interpret these numbers and ask himself, *Do I do nothing to try to get the number lower? Do I take a shot of insulin? Do I exercise?* In other words, an act is backed by intention. If the person intended to take a nap, he would take one action (take insulin). Intending to take a walk would lead to another action (or nonaction in terms of taking medication).

The third type of knowledge evidenced in the text and talk of diabetes is bodily knowledge, a type of knowledge based on physical sensations. Like the terms *episteme* and *techne,* the concept of bodily knowledge is contested, but in rhetorical theory these definitions generally follow feminist critics such as

Grosz (1994) in defining bodies as changeable rather than static.[6] The definition of bodily knowledge that I use here draws on a tacit understanding as
well, but is more similar to Sauer's (2003) definition of pit sense: "an embodied
sensory knowledge derived from site-specific practice in a particular working
environment" (p. 219).

In other words, pit sense requires what one of my focus group participants defined as "finding what works for you." For people with diabetes, the
sensations that accompany hypoglycemia, blood sugar levels that dip to dangerously low levels, or hyperglycemia, high levels of blood sugar, would be
examples of this type of knowledge. To use this sense requires the ability to
apply scientific principles to local situations. For people with diabetes, this
might include applying the medical knowledge about the symptoms of an
episode of low blood sugar to that person's individual experience of low blood
sugar. Like the miners that Sauer (2003) studies, the environment in which
my diabetic participants employed bodily knowledge is risky. A person has
the immediate danger of blood sugar levels dropping too low and potentially
passing out and perhaps moving into seizures or a coma if treatment is not
quick. There is also the long-term specter of serious complications if blood
sugars remain at high levels for too long over time.

Kerri Morrone Sparling, a well-known diabetic blogger, gives a powerful
example of working in this dangerous environment on her blog *Six Until Me*.
One of her posts is a video of herself experiencing a real-time hypoglycemic
episode.

> So here's a fun one. Um, I'm 54. Not years—blood sugar is 54. And instead
> of vlogging about what I wanted to vlog about, I'm waiting impatiently for
> my blood sugar to come up. And this is one of those weird times where I
> can sort of speak coherently, but I don't know, the words, I can actually see
> them like, like typewriter type going across my eyes and, you know, at least
> across my mind. . . . (Sparling, 2009, seconds 11–36)

---

6. Feminist theorists such as Harding (1991) and Haraway (1992) have also argued that
knowledge production needs to take the situated view of individuals into account. Rhetoricians of health and medicine pick up Haraway's (1991) suspicion of technologically mediated
embodiment. For example, Mary Lay's 2000 analysis is primarily concerned with how direct-
entry midwives communicate women's embodied knowledge within discursive spaces that place
a high value on scientific knowledge. She makes a distinction between technological and what
she referred to as embodied knowledge, but she also likens embodied knowledge to experien-
tial knowledge. Similarly, Owens (2009) draws a distinction in women's birthing experiences
through an analysis of birth plans. She argues that the increase in technological and scientific
knowledge is accompanied by a parallel trust in that knowledge.

As Kerri talks through this bodily sensation, the viewers can hear her speech alternate between slowing down and increasing in its pace. She slurs a bit as if she were drunk. Viewers can, in other words, see the embodied experience of the low blood sugar she is experiencing. This experience of "*doing* hypoglycemia," as Mol and Law (2004) argue, "is not only a matter of *knowing* it by measuring it from the outside, feeling it from the inside, or some combination of the two" (p. 48; emphasis in original). Doing hypoglycemia requires intervention. Therefore, bodily knowledge of the sensations of a low blood sugar is a form of knowledge that impacts what people with diabetes do.

Through a series of vignettes of people with diabetes and medical practitioners talking about hypoglycemia, Mol and Law (2004) suggest that hypoglycemia is "done" through three types of interventions—counteracting, avoiding, and producing. People with diabetes counteract low blood sugar by eating. One of the people Mol and Law (2004) discuss describes waking up in the middle of the night with symptoms of a low blood sugar—shivering and sweating. She gets up and immediately eats something. A diabetic nurse they interviewed describes an elderly woman patient who is so afraid of having a low blood sugar that she would constantly overeat and, therefore, avoid one. Producing hypoglycemia may seem counterintuitive since people with diabetes are taught to avoid both hypoglycemia and hyperglycemia to try to keep their blood sugars in a target range, but, in fact, many people with diabetes use what the medical community calls "tight control" in order to reduce the likelihood of complications in the future. This is particularly true for people on intensive insulin therapy, which requires multiple insulin injections per day or the use of an insulin pump. As such, it requires people to pay much closer attention to their blood sugar numbers throughout the day—not only in terms of administering insulin to themselves more frequently but also monitoring their blood sugar levels more frequently throughout the day. Someone not on intensive therapy might take an oral medication once a day or an insulin injection once a day and, therefore, would not need to test blood sugar levels as frequently. People with such tight control, however, also run a greater risk of *producing* hypoglycemic episodes.

During these hypoglycemic episodes, most people experience a subset of the many symptoms of low blood sugar.[7] One person on the TuDiabetes forums said, for example: "For me, when my blood-sugar first begins to get

---

7. Some people have hypoglycemia unawareness. This condition occurs more frequently in people who frequently have low blood glucose episodes (which can cause a person to stop sensing the early warning signs of hypoglycemia), have had diabetes for a long time, and/or people who tightly control their diabetes (ADA, 2015).

too low I usually feel weak and tired. A shaky, unstable feeling sets in that is usually accompanied by a 'panic' feeling." Members of this community often compare notes, checking with each other about typical symptoms and more atypical ones they have experienced such as visual hallucinations or muscle spasms. The Conversation Map discussed in chapter 1 also provides an example of pit sense in this environment. One activity in the game involves a discussion of high and low blood sugar symptoms that are outlined on playing cards. Daisy, a certified diabetes educator I interviewed, handed out these cards to her group of patients. Each card listed a physical sensation linked to high blood sugar or low blood sugar, such as shaking, irritability, or blurred vision. Daisy asked each person to guess whether the symptom was related to high blood sugar levels or low blood sugar levels. As Daisy led the group through this exercise, she stressed that these reactions are individual: "Everyone will not experience the same ones." This statement then led to a side discussion by the participants of the specific symptoms they experienced.

Knowledge developed from physical signs or sensations of the body, therefore, is extremely important. To paraphrase Nikki, understanding the disease is important, but only because that knowledge makes it easier to attend to the body, but not just the diabetic body writ large—the specific body. In my interview transcripts, this physically situated knowledge was often expressed with the phrase *for me*. An example comes from the following excerpt from a focus group that consisted of one person with type 2 diabetes (Mary) and three people with type 1 (Grace, David, and Connie). When the participants discuss their roles in their own health care teams, Mary distinguished her experience from the others:

> MARY: I have an endocrinologist, he's also an internist, so it's the same person that I go see. [. . .] But like I said, it's a little different *for me* [emphasis added] because again as a type 2 it's always easy to forget, you know, and say, "life goes on."

David uses the phrase in his definition of "control."

> DAVID: I think *for me* [emphasis added] being in good control, I guess I can see two sides of it. Not that I like to use the scare tactics of "you're going to lose a leg and you're going to lose your eye sight," but I really value my legs and my eye sight, so I think keeping that in check as a typical modality of not taking care of my disease is pretty motivating.

This attention to bodily knowledge was much more prevalent in the patient texts than in the provider interviews or organizational website texts.

Representations of bodily knowledge, or pit sense, do exist in provider texts, but they are not as easily identifiable as examples of epistemic knowledge and techne. Examples of bodily knowledge on the websites are limited to general patient scenarios based on the treatment and issues of type 1 and type 2 diabetes, as in the following scenarios from the website of the U.S. Department of Veteran Affairs:

> **Scenario #1:** Bob D., age 49, has type 2 diabetes. For the past seven years, he and his doctor have worked to control his blood sugar levels with diet and diabetes pills. Recently, Bob's control has been getting worse, so his doctor said that Bob might have to start insulin shots. But first, they agreed that Bob would try an exercise program to improve control. After 3 months of sticking to his exercise plan, Bob returned to the doctor to check his blood sugar. It was near the normal range, but the doctor knew a single blood test only showed Bob's control at that time. It didn't say much about Bob's overall blood sugar control. The doctor sent a sample of Bob's blood to the lab for an A1C test to learn how well Bob's blood sugar had been controlled, on average, for the past few months. The A1C test showed that Bob's control had improved. With the A1C results, Bob and his doctor had proof that the exercise program was working. The test results also helped Bob know that he could make a difference in his blood sugar control.
>
> **Scenario #2:** Nine-year-old Lisa J. and her parents were proud that she could do her own insulin shots and urine tests. Her doctor advised her to begin a routine of two shots a day and regular blood glucose checks [. . .] (U.S. Department of Veteran Affairs, 2013, How Does it Help Diabetes Control?)

Along with providing a general scenario that cannot capture individual bodily knowledge, these scenarios share an emphasis on certain knowledge typically attributed to episteme in Bob's case and techne in Lisa's case. The conversation Bob had with his doctor about his exercise habits does not appear to have been persuasive, but the A1C test result is. The reader assumes that Bob is, in fact, sticking to the agreed-upon exercise plan. Rather than being satisfied with Bob's report about his activities and the normal blood glucose test performed by the patient, however, the doctor questions both of these bodily experiences and chooses to rely on the certainty of the A1C value produced by a lab. As the scenario indicates, the body exists as a record for someone else to interpret: a record of blood sugar readings or changes in eye health and blood pressure readings as described in Step 3 of the NDEP web page. Therefore, the episteme of the doctor is held in higher regard than bodily knowledge.

The following text excerpt from the Joslin Diabetes Center website separates the person from body sensations as well:

Remember, your eyes can become damaged without your knowing it, as the damage can occur in areas that do not affect vision and you often feel no pain. Only careful eye examinations at regular intervals will detect the damage. If you have type 1 diabetes, it's a good idea to have your eyes examined by an eye doctor expert in diabetes care at least once a year. Call your eye doctor's office if you experience any of the following symptoms:

- sudden loss of vision
- severe eye pain
- the sensation that a curtain is coming down over your eyes
- black or red floating spots in your vision.
- distortion or waviness of straight lines

Your eye doctor will want to see you right away.[8]

In phrases such as "your eyes can become damaged" and "have your eyes examined by an eye doctor expert in diabetes care," the body is depicted as separate from the patient. Obviously, bodily knowledge does come into play in these texts, but only as certain and objective signs from which to glean information. Furthermore, the texts privilege a binary relationship between body and disease rather than a self-care that pays attention to the language we use to express our experiences and our health or illness and an interconnectedness with others, as in a feminist perspective on relational autonomy and a feminist ethic of care.[9] Relational autonomy represents a range of perspectives with the shared conviction "that persons are socially embedded and that agents' identities are formed within the context of social relationships" (Heid, 2006, p. 48). Such relational autonomy understands individual actions in the context of social practices (Jaggar, 1991).[10] Within conversations about patient agency, one of those relationships is between the person with diabetes and the person's body.

---

8. Copyright © 2016 by Joslin Diabetes Center. All rights reserved. Reprinted with permission from www.joslin.org.

9. See Emmons (2010), *Black Dogs and Blue Words*.

10. See Carol Gilligan's and Nel Noddings's extensive work on feminist ethics of care as well as Catriona Mackenzie and Natalie Stolar's 2000 edited collection *Relational Autonomy: Feminist Perspectives on Autonomy, Agency, and the Social Self*.

ACTIVATING AGENCY

A problem with seeing agency through such a terministic screen (Burke, 1966) is that a patient is always conscribed to learn a specialized knowledge or perform an act as a mechanical or habitual repetition of the thing that is to be learned. Such a rote view of learning is apparent in the phrase being used in many medical situations, the *active* patient, which typically denotes a patient who is a lay expert about his or her disease. Different disease communities characterize the active patient differently. For example, according to the Cancer Support Community, in the cancer community an active patient is one who is informed, takes action, and connects with others. In the HIV/AIDS community, being active has been characterized in four ways: "the patient as *manager of his illness*, the *empowerment* of patients, the *science-wise* patient and the *experimenter*" (Barbot, 2006, p. 538; emphasis in original). Within the framework of the Chronic Care Model, an expert diabetes patient is called *activated* rather than active. The concept is meant to be a positive move away from viewing patients as passive objects, but Mol (2008) argued that it is intimately linked to the concept of patient choice. From a viewpoint that prioritizes choice, patients are placed in a binary relationship with their disease: the patient is the subject and choice is the object. Mol cautions that in health care, active patients are not "subjects of choice" but "subjects of all kinds of activities" (Mol, 2008, p. 8) because the focus is (or should be) on what they do in a broader network rather than their desire or will to do something in a space in which just the patient and disease exist. In the Chronic Model of Care, the agency of the patient/agent is seen primarily as a top-down process that reflects the concern that Mol voiced. In this process, knowledge is produced and given to patients by medical experts and authorities.

Used in diabetes discourse, the term also picks up echoes of techne and the definition of patient agency as taking actions to successfully control blood sugar. However, the way people with diabetes use the various types of knowledge available to them suggests that the action here is moving between types of knowledge—episteme, techne, and bodily knowledge—as they acquire, use, create, and share knowledge. Much in the way that Campbell (2005) proposed learning rhetoric by studying, training, and experiencing, people with diabetes draw on episteme, techne, and pit sense. This triad, unlike the narratives of progress discussed in chapter 1, is not related to a linear progression. These three things can be done in one order or another or they could be done simultaneously. These oscillations require rethinking the linear and hierarchal approach to knowledge acquisition, use, production, and sharing as a *way* of knowing through metis. *Metis*, a Greek term often defined as wisdom, skill, or craft, is associated with Odysseus in his travails during and after the Trojan War as well as with Prometheus's skill in stealing fire from the gods (Detienne & Vernant, 1978).[11] Although metis had been an under-explored concept for quite some time, contemporary scholars are finding the concept useful for a number of projects. Kopelson (2003) uses it to describe pedagogical attempts to counter student resistance in composition classes, and Popham (2014) suggests it is an appropriate frame from which to understand multidisciplinary identities in her examination of the mental health electronic records of juveniles. Miller (2000) and Ballif (1998) also critique the traditional rhetoric of techne, proposing alternatives of metis for the practice of technical communication.[12]

The connection metis has to "making do" in a given situation is a fruitful one for the permanently liminal nature of diabetes. At once flexible and practical, metis is "full of reversals and thus demanding resourcefulness" (Dolmage, 2009, p. 6). It can deal with "whatever comes up" (Detienne & Vernant, 1978, p. 22). It also helps move past a linear sense of knowledge acquisition and application taken up by medical professionals and the texts created for people with diabetes, as Bragg's (2004) definition of metis as cunning intelligence suggests: "in contrast to the linear progress of rational thought, [metis] never goes forward in a straight line but is always weaving from side to side and looping back on itself" (p. 32).[13] Finally, metis separates a person's actions from prudent actions, which has obvious benefits in dis-articulating subjectivities of blame and shame from people with diabetes. Unlike phronesis, which implies acting with prudence and has connections to the goals of "truth" and wisdom, metis "has the freedom to be less moral and seeks an isolated result." (Dolmage, 2009, p. 11).[14] In diabetes self-management, practi-

---

11. Schryer et al. (2005) remind us that treatises like Isocrates's *Against the Sophists* and Hippocrates's *Ancient Medicine, The Art, and The Oath* indicate that "techne also meant something like a cunning set of flexible strategies that partially controlled human or natural events" (p. 239). Recent scholarship (Atwill, 1998; Cahn, 1989; Dunne, 1993; Papillion, 1995; Roochnik, 1996) has also provided new insights into the nature of techne as akin to metis, or what Schryer et al. (2005) call "savvy knowledge" (p. 234).

12. In writing of metis and a postmodern form of invention, Miller (2000) ties metis to hunting and a worldview concerned with individual cases rather than universal knowledge. Ballif (1998) associates metis with navigation: "Because the human condition is often characterized by change and the ungovernable forces of nature and fate, *mêtis* equips the possessor with the ways and means to negotiate the flux" (p. 65).

13. Moeller & McAllister (2002) suggest that techne involves cunning and is "full of trickery" (p. 185) as well.

14. Phronesis, roughly translated as prudence, however, is typically linked with episteme (or scientific knowledge) and aligned with the goal of "truth" and wisdom. It is also linked to virtue. Aristotle argued that phronesis allows us to pursue a goal, but virtue tells us how to pur-

cal wisdom would lead to an excellent decision. If a blood sugar was too high, the "excellent" decision would be to take action that results in lowering the blood sugar number. As such, action is not contextualized but is assumed to be tied to an overarching definition of what is *right*: a definition intertwined with the biomedical definition of compliance and narratives of progress. Metis dis-articulates virtue from notions of knowledge and situates *truth*.

People with diabetes use metis to situate truth through wayfinding, troubleshooting, and experimentation. *Wayfinding* refers to the series of things a person knows and does in order to get from one place to another (Carpman & Grant, 2006). In an architectural sense, this may refer to how a person navigates an urban landscape. In digital environments it refers to how people search online. "Finding what works for you," a phrase so many people with diabetes use when talking about advice they would give another diabetic, sounds very much like wayfinding, especially if we think of it as a form of troubleshooting or knowledge use rather than knowledge acquisition. It is complicated and requires tracing numerous complicated systems to find the trouble. Is my blood sugar high because I'm getting sick? No, I don't have a fever. Was it something I ate? Unlikely, I only had a salad and apple for lunch. The following excerpt shows such troubleshooting language. In giving advice to a diabetic new to insulin pump technology, one TuDiabetes community member suggested the following:

> Speaking of pump sites, don't feel bad about trying other infusion sets and different lengths of tubing and different cannula lengths. Find what works best for you, and sometimes that means having different sets for different areas. For example, I like the contact detach for my arms and the inset everywhere else, but I'll tolerate the inset on my arms if I have to.

Another person advises another member new to the community:

> I'm sure others will chime in w/ slightly different methods that may also be helpful—you'll just have to do some trial and error to ultimately find what works best for you.

Figuring out complicated adjustments to insulin therapy to account for individual differences that no arithmetic formula can account for, people with diabetes clearly experiment on themselves through trial and error, as the

---

sue it. Aristotle implied that the practically wise person will make "excellent decisions" (Warne, 2006, p. 6).

TuDiabetes community member stated. To find what works best, diabetics become their own guinea pigs, as evident in other posts as well, such as the following:

> It's taken 5 years to accept that I am my own experiment. The doctors/educators/et.al. can only make suggestions. They have a lot of knowledge that they learned through other diabetics and books but the actual doing of life is going to be different for me than it will be for another diabetic so I use their input as a guideline and not the Bible.

As my focus group participant Nikki further noted, no one diabetic is the same as the next. Interestingly, this n-of-1 mindset has been picked up by members of the medical community, if not by medical professionals specifically focusing on diabetes. N-of-1—or single subject studies—clinical trials, use the individual patient as the unit of observation to study the efficacy or side effect of an intervention with the goal of determining the best option for that individual patient (Lillie et al., 2011). At the same time, people with diabetes have used the gold standard of medicine, the clinical trial, for their own experimentation, as suggested by this comment from Elliott in one of my focus groups:

> You know, a place that I've learned that's kind of nontraditional is in diabetic trials. For most of my life I have tried to do diabetic trials whenever possible, and it's amazing . . . it's the unusual stuff you hear during the trials that later becomes gospel in the diabetic community, and I find that to be a place that I go to find information.

In fact, members of the TuDiabetes community have an entire forum dedicated to information about ongoing clinical trials, and threads like the following excerpt indicate that the community regularly participates in these trials:

> ORIGINAL POST: Has anyone done any clinical trials for new onset or recent onset type 1 that preserves beta cells, like abate? I was wondering if anyone did it and if they thought it was not so bad, if it worked, any info? I was thinking to put my daughter in one, I would love to stay in the honeymoon.
> REPLY 1: Check out joshualevy.com "Cures for Diabetes." He lists all the trials, what phase they are in, and has links to the research papers. You will be able to go to one web site and get tons of information. Good luck. . . .

REPLY 2: have you ever looked into faustman? faustmanlab.org. It looks
hugely promising and I want to get involved in this. (on the cure front.)
REPLY 3: Faustman is very promising but it's a bit behind other ongoing trials
that have pretty solid results.

The lengthy responses the original comment received about clinical trials
would indicate that people with diabetes are not only interested in experimentation on themselves as a way to access cutting-edge treatment, but also
as a way to gain (and share) knowledge. In fact, they not only gain knowledge through this participation, they participate in evaluating the rigor of the
scientific studies themselves on the forum, much in the same way that Paige
evaluated the guidelines from different expert organizations. A particular clinical trial has gained a good amount of attention in the TuDiabetes community, that of Dr. Denise Faustman, director of the Immunobiology Laboratory
at the Massachusetts General Hospital (MGH) and an associate professor of
medicine at Harvard Medical School. Faustman's clinical trial focuses on the
efficacy of the BCG vaccine (the bacille Calmette-Guerin vaccine used for
tuberculosis) for reversing long-term type 1 diabetes. The following comment
was posted on a discussion forum on the website in response to a thread with
a video interview posted on TuDiabetes with Dr. Faustman on July 24, 2014:

> The big elephant in the room to me was why did it take 10 years and 12 mil-
> lion dollars to run a Phase 1 trial on 6 (yes, six) people? The positive take-
> away was that things should be starting to move a bit into Phase 2 where
> they'll be analyzing outcomes of different dosages on different folks, how-
> ever, she still needs another 8 million dollars to reach the 25 million goal,
> so I'm not sure how quickly it will move forward. There don't appear to be
> any risks and BCG has a 100-year safety profile. FDA wasn't listed as an
> obstacle. No, she didn't discuss when Phase 3 would be, though I had read
> that Phase 2 will take around 4-6 years. The thing that has me so baffled is
> the timetable of it all.

To make the claim that Faustman's research is questionable, the person evaluates timelines, safety, research design, and funding. Traditionally these are
the concerns of a scientist rather than a patient. For example, in a grant proposal submitted to the National Institutes of Health (NIH), a researcher needs
to include a narrative about the research design, information regarding the
safety and protection of the people participating in the research study and
approval of the institution's Institutional Review Board (IRB), a budget, a list

of current and pending support, and a description of facilities, equipment, and other resources. Once submitted, the grant goes through a peer review process. According to the NIH Office of Extramural Research, the first level of review is carried out by a Scientific Review Group (SRG), which includes scientists with expertise in relevant scientific disciplines and current research areas. After this review, the proposal moves to a second-level review, which is performed, by the Institute and Center (IC) National Advisory Councils or Boards. These councils include both scientific and public representatives. The final funding decisions are made by the IC Directors (NIH, 2014). The people involved in discussions of research projects like Dr. Faustman's are, in effect, participating in a similar, if more open, peer review process of research protocols. As such, people with diabetes interpret meaning rather than absorb knowledge or memorize new information, as they are represented to be doing in the ADA and NDEP texts I discussed earlier in the chapter.

The final way people with diabetes wayfind, experiment, and troubleshoot is through hacking their own bodies and the technologies they use. Although the participants of my study did not mention hacking or other acts of metis, as the opening of this chapter suggests, the online community of people with diabetes are active hackers. One of the most notable instances occurred in 2013 when Jason Adams, a business-development executive, developed a way to monitor his eight-year-old daughter's blood-sugar levels. Nightscout, a system created by Adams and a group of software engineers (many with diabetic children), uploads data to the Internet, which lets parents monitor their child's blood sugar on devices like smartphones and smartwatches when the child is away from home. Jay Radcliffe performed troubleshooting in a different way when he biohacked his own insulin pump. According to a 2014 *Reuters* report, in 2011 Radcliffe demonstrated the technique at the Def Con hacking conference in Las Vegas for remotely hacking into the Medtronic insulin pump he used through the wireless communications system the pump uses. At the conference, Radcliffe stated that the approach could have been used to deliver lethal doses of insulin to patients.[15]

Both Adams and Radcliffe not only created new technologies and new knowledge, but both shared this knowledge with others. Nightscout is basically CGM in the cloud. It is an open source, DIY project that allows people real-time access to a Dexcom G4 CGM from web browsers via smartphones, computers, tablets, and the Pebble Smartwatch. The goal of the project is to allow remote monitoring of the type 1 diabetic's glucose level using existing

---

15. According to the same report, in 2011 Medtronic hired security consultants to review the safety of its insulin pumps. The company found more vulnerabilities in the devices, which they said were also potentially lethal.

monitoring devices. According to a story in *The Wall Street Journal,* Kristin Derichsweiler downloaded the software to help her 15-year-old son manage his diabetes. One day while she was at work, she noticed his blood sugar dropping to dangerously low levels. When he failed to answer the phone, she rushed home. Her son had become unresponsive and needed assistance with getting juice to drink to restore proper sugar levels.[16] Radcliff went so far as to identify himself as a spokesperson for other people with diabetes, announcing in a blog post after the Def Con conference, "Emerging technologies in the medical world are often ill-equipped for the dangers that the interconnected world faces, and we need spokespeople to draw attention to these dangers. As a diabetic, who depends on these interconnected devices to live, I find myself as an advocate in this arena" (Radcliffe, 2014).

Other smaller hacks happen every day that evidence both knowledge creation and sharing via metis. In 2013, blogger Kerri Morrone Sparling was invited to present at the International Diabetes Federation World Congress, an umbrella organization of over 230 national diabetes associations in 170 countries and territories that represents the interests of people with diabetes and those at risk (IDF, 2015). One of the things she talked about was the Dexcom-in-a-Glass hack (Sparling, 2011). She and other people that use Dexcom's continuous blood glucose monitoring system place the device in a glass by their bedside at night. The glass makes the alarms the meter gives for low and high blood sugars easier to hear when sleeping. Tom, who you met in the introduction, talked about another life hack:

> This is at least a two-part answer. The first part is getting the receiver to take readings again: you can either find Stop Sensor in your menu, or wait until the receiver tells you that the 7-day period has expired (and it stops taking readings on its own). After that sensor has stopped, go back to your menu and select Start Sensor. After another two-hour period, you can calibrate (by entering two fingerstick results) and continue on, with the receiver believing you're using a fresh sensor, when it really is the one you were already wearing.

Whether finding what works or making something work better, through metis patients perform agency through the act of situational meaning making, enacting the making and recirculating of meaning as they perform agency through articulating and re-articulating epistemic, practical, and bodily

---

16. Since this time, Dexcom has integrated a similar function into its continuous glucose monitoring system. It can be argued that Nightscout played a role in getting this technology developed.

knowledge. Diabetics thus act much like makers in maker spaces. They are inventors, designers, and tinkerers. Maker spaces, like group patient appointment spaces and online patient communities, are creative spaces in which people gather to create, invent, and learn. If agency is a negotiation or process that takes place in a network of materials and relations in such spaces, agency can emerge and be performed in the collaborative spaces of diabetes care. Including metis as a possible way of making meaning—along with epistemic knowledge, techne, and bodily knowledge—helps erode the boundary between this and that and make room for a practice of articulation that moves these settings themselves into a constellation rather than a binary.

CHAPTER 4

Shifting Subjectivities

Attributed and Interactional Expertise

> Think of me as a Shiva, a many-armed and legged body with one foot on
> brown soil, one on white, one in straight society, one in the gay world, the
> man's world, the woman's, one limb in the literary world, another in the work-
> ing class, the socialist, and the occult worlds. A sort of spider woman hanging
> by one thin strand of web
>
> —G. Anzaldúa, *Borderlands La Frontera: The New Mestiza*

IDENTITIES OF expert patients are largely formed around the oscillating articulations people with diabetes make with different types of knowledge in terms
of the individual—a diabetic's experience in becoming a subject matter expert.
This form of expertise is expressed through a mastery of material, whether the
material is more theoretical, practical, or physical. A clear example of such a
subject matter expert is evident in online discussion forums when people self-
report their medical situations:

> last night my dexcom cgm went bonkers. the High alarm kept going off w/
> an UP direction arrow. i did a finger stick; my BG was 145 (pretty good) so
> i recalibrated my receiver. then, w/in 1/2 hour, my alarm went off again, this
> time LOW. i did another finger stick; BG 125; no problem. so i recalibrated
> again. this went on all night at least 5 to 6 times. it kept waking me up when
> the alarms went off. my husband is a light sleeper and the alarms were driv-
> ing him crazy. also, i kept having to use up my test strips, which are very
> expensive. this morning i ripped the darn thing off and put on a new one to
> start a sensor "session." i must have hit a blood vessel, b/c blood started com-
> ing out around the sensor. so, i ripped this one off, which was also expensive
> b/c i use the NEXCARE tape over the transmitter. next, i put another sensor
> on, and i hit a nerve. oooow what pain!!!! so i took that one off. now, i am
> on my 3rd sensor. finally, w/ this one i got lucky; the sensor felt comfortable

and i was ready to go for the 2 hour wait period to calibrate with the 2 BG #s. when the "session" period was over, i calibrated the 1st BG#, which was 194. then i did my 2nd finger stick and the BG# was 176; the HIGH alarm went off. what should i do? i called dexcom and asked them what to do. i think that i finally have reached success, but i probably won't know until later on in the day.[1]

This particular individual shows expertise in a variety of ways. First, the person's description of the actions taken (techne) when she responds to the alarm indicates that she knows how to use a complex medical device. The characterizations of a blood sugar of 145 as "pretty good" and 125 as "no problem" also indicate that she is knowledgeable about the range of blood sugar levels that are desirable. Finally, after taking several sensors off her body, she goes through the physical (bodily) process of calibrating the instrument.

Subject-matter mastery, however, is not the only form of expertise people with diabetes enact through subjectivities of expert patients. In liminal, collective spaces, attributed expertise (Hartelius, 2011) becomes apparent because it is established through the relationship with an audience. In other words, to be experts, people must persuade others that they are. As Hartelius (2011) describes, "It is an *attributed* state of being-with-others in which one's performance is evaluated irrespective of so-called 'real knowledge'" (p. 4; emphasis in original). This type of expertise has a great deal in common with the dynamic nature of agency:

> What is unmistakably present in the live speaking situation is an Other [i.e., an audience], someone who may resist, disagree, disapprove, humiliate—or approve, appreciate, empathize, and applaud. . . . To produce kinetic energy, performance requires a relationship between two entities who will *attribute* agency to each other. (Miller, 2007, p. 149; emphasis in original)

ATTRIBUTING EXPERTISE

People with diabetes attribute expertise to each other in a number of ways. One way is through identification (Burke, 1950). As Burke states, identification brings people together, but one of the reasons we feel the need to come together is that we do not only experience separateness but we feel guilty

---

1. Diabetics are encouraged to verify the number that appears on the continuous glucose monitor (CGM) before taking actions that could severely impact their immediate health if that number is wrong.

about the differences between ourselves and others. Therefore, we look for things we share with others to overcome this guilt as well as separateness. Amy, one of the pharmacists interviewed, tells a story that reflects this guilt:

> I had two patients with one maybe in denial . . . maybe a newly diagnosed . . . maybe they're in denial they think they're so sick now because they have diabetes and it's horrible and then you start talking about, oh, "what's your A1C?" or, "what's a high blood sugar you've had." Then suddenly someone comes up and says, "well the highest I've had is like 400 something." And the other person goes, "Oh, maybe I'm not so bad because my high was only 180." It isn't the end of the world. Sure, that person with the 400 blood sugar shouldn't be that way, but you know it gives the other person the perspective, yeah okay, puts their disease in a little bit different perspective.

The denial Amy talks about the first person experiencing (the person with a blood sugar of 180) is a type of guilt based on the perception that this number is too high. In other words, there is a difference between this patient and a nondiabetic person with normal blood sugar levels. To overcome such division, we often look for ways in which our interests, attitudes, values, experiences, perceptions, and material properties are shared with others, or could appear to be shared. For a person with diabetes, once the person is given an opportunity to identify with someone more similar and with numbers that are even higher, the guilt lessens. Tom sums this up well in part of his response to a question about the value of group sessions.

> A group setting of maybe four or five people would certainly be good, if the group was on a pretty similar educational level as far as their diabetic education, and then maybe similar time in terms of their disease progression. It may not be great if you had people that were newly diagnosed with people that have been treating it for quite a while. Having some commonality or some range of comfort or educational level or just diabetic education. It would help everybody to progress equally.

For Tom, similarities in education levels and disease progression smooth out ripples of difference. Providers recognize this identification as well:

> EMILY (PHARMACIST): I would say I've noticed an advantage [to group classes] when I have more people in here versus less. When there's a group they're all diabetics. So, you know, I start talking about something and then someone says, "oh yeah, I had this experience," and the other

people in the class take more from what that person can say than if I were to say it.

KATHY (PHARMACIST): Sometimes they start talking amongst themselves about issues that they've had or they might bring up. "Oh, I need a knee replacement; I go to this doctor." "Oh, do you like that doctor?" "Yeah, he's a good doctor."

One of the more light-hearted ways this identification occurs online is with the "You Know You're Diabetic When" discussion thread on the TuDiabetes website. This thread is one of the more popular ones and regularly reappears in the conversation online. Responses are usually humorous:

You know you're a diabetic when you get a giggle out of being able to say "I woke up high." Who else gets to say that?

When you become adept at multiplying and dividing by 18.

You know you're a diabetic when after finding test strips all over your house you find one outside or in the super market and you feel obligated to pick it up!

But members of an online community identify with each other through more serious similarities as well, as the following excerpts in response to a question about what makes a person online a credible resource show.

NIKKI: Oh, this is terrible. This is terrible, but I'll admit to it. I'll cop out and admit that I do this. And if it's some kind of great control advice and somebody is trying to tell me that I can achieve great control if I do x, y, or z, I tend to go to their profile and on the profile there is a list of questions and you can list what your A1C is, and I go in and look at their A1C. You know, because I want to know just how credible is this and does it really work, you know?

PAIGE: Even though you're dealing with avatars rather than people in many cases, or you only know somebody's first name, it's clear if you hang out on the site long enough who the intelligent, well informed, medically educated are on there both by the internal consistency in their posts, the kinds of things that they reference, the kinds of discussions that they participate in. And over time I've pretty much gotten to know whose advice I can trust on there.

In looking at how lay people evaluate technical products based on online reviews, Mackiewicz (2010) recognized a relationship between credibility and trustworthiness, finding that trustworthiness generates credibility and "rises out of character and good intentions, as well as knowledge (i.e., expertise)" (p. 7). Reviewers became trustworthy by making assertions directly about their expertise and conveying their expertise by employing specialized terminology and establishing a reputation. In online diabetes communities, a comparable relationship is valued, and reputation, trustworthiness, and credibility are established through analogous lived experiences.

Peer Mentors and the Wisdom of the Crowd

Identification or sameness often sets up a peer mentoring relationship for people with diabetes. Medical providers describe how patients mentor each other in their collaborative education spaces. Amy's description of an interaction in one of their group educational sessions illustrates this:

> AMY: I would say that an advantage of the group classes I've noticed when I have more people in here versus less, when there's a group they're all diabetics. So, you know, I start talking about something and then someone says, "oh yeah, I had this experience" and the other people in the class I think take more from what that person can say than if I were to say it. Because they know it's coming from another diabetic so they kind of start to bond over their experiences.

By "bonding" and "having the same experience," as Amy says, diabetics are identifying with each other. Much like what Mackiewicz (2010) found for online reviews, the process of identification for people with diabetes is helped along by a person's trustworthiness:

> SCOTT: Yeah, I've had that [happen] too. They can learn from each other though, like you were saying. Maybe they retain some of it more or actually use some of the knowledge a little bit better if someone who actually has it has done it—if they say it versus one of us, just sitting there lecturing people. We had two ladies in here and it was around diet issues and they were, you know, the one lady was saying how she struggled with, I forget exactly what the food was that she was eating that was unhealthy. Then the other lady said, "Well, have you tried this? It's a really good food and it's healthier for you, you know? I eat it." And it's something we [the pharmacists] would recommend, and I think you know sometimes if you have that experience. You know, at least diet, it seems like

it is something a lot of people struggle with—changing their diet. And
when they hear somebody else that has diabetes likes something, maybe
they're willing to try it or eat.

Interestingly, one of the side effects of identification and peer mentoring relationships is that people with diabetes use their similarities to set up differences that enable a person to claim and be recognized as *more expert* than the
person asking for advice, information, or support. Sara offers advice based
on her own expertise and bodily knowledge of diabetes as well as her experience as a person with asthma, for authority. She says, "Well, as an asthmatic,
I KNOW what steroids do to blood sugars, and it is hateful." Such direct language discursively establishes her authority as an expert patient. Another person indicates a position of authority from a past personal experience with
eating disorders.

> I can tell you from having an eating disorder that not eating will send the
> numbers soaring. You need a diabetic class thru your hospital or clinic. I am
> taking a six-month class as I don't eat all the food groups and having prob-
> lems eating. It's okay to validate what you are feeling but there is so much
> more to life than this. I control my diabetes; it does not control me.

This individual is comfortable giving advice that might otherwise come from
a medical professional. A doctor, for instance, might engage a patient to see a
nutritionist if they were having trouble with diet changes or weight. As such,
this writer "can tell"—a much more expert position than one that suggests or
advises. The other expert relies on questioning the person being responded
to. Even Tom, who specifically noted the value of similarities with another
diabetic in group appointments, also recognizes the value of a less-equal, mentoring relationship:

> On the converse, there may be some people that have had it for a while that
> do enjoy serving in more of an educational role, or the "I'll put my arm
> around you and tell you what I know and help you along with the progres-
> sion of the disease."

This imbalanced relationship also comes out in what Ken, a provider participant who is also diabetic, called the wisdom of the crowd. The following two
excerpts come from one focus group.

> ELLIOTT: I probably trust folks the least probably because I've heard over
> time virtually every harebrained idea out there. I think if I hear it four or

five times then I might start to pay attention to it. I just don't believe that there's going to be a significant cure or a significant change that's going to occur on TuDiabetes that I'm not going to know from some other place, so I guess it's verification from other places.

Other participants picked up on this type of attribution as well:

CONNIE: You know what, usually if I get some information, I'll go right to a search and I'll search and look at 10 different sources before I make a decision whether or not I believe it or not. And I go to as many different sources as I can find. I do that with everything.

GRACE: I'm the same way.

What Ken refers to as the wisdom of the crowd is a form of social proof. As a means of persuasion, social proofs are useful when people are uncertain about a particular course of action, such as whether or not to follow a particular diet. When they are uncertain, they will look to others to help guide their decision making and actions (Caldini, 1984). In looking to others, people are particularly interested in what their peers are doing because they identify with them, but this also puts the people being *looked to* into positions of authority.

People with diabetes also use this wisdom to question providers' advice. Paige, a focus group participant, said,

I think that the way that you get empowered in modern times is to come to your medical appointment with as much information as possible and the Internet makes it much easier to have alternative sources of information about things. And sometimes things will work that a doctor or a certified diabetes educator wouldn't necessarily recommend. I mean, I have met on the Internet a large number of people who are having much lower carb diets than the so-called recommendations for diabetics, and the medical profession as a whole doesn't seem to be acknowledging the value of that, but it works for a ton of people. So, if you know something like that you go in better armed than if you say, "I'm just going to do exactly what you say, doctor."[2]

Paige enacts her expertise by comparing information that is accepted by the diabetes patient community she belongs to online to the guidance that the general provider community gives about low carbohydrate diets for people

---

2. It is interesting to note that before the discovery of insulin people with diabetes were basically treated using what was called a starvation diet, which would have excluded carbohydrates.

with diabetes.[3] Traditionally medical professionals have advised people with diabetes not to use such diets because insulin and oral medications act on carbohydrate: A diabetic determines the amount of insulin to give himself based on the grams of carbohydrate he is about to eat. Doctors also prescribe oral medications partially based on the amount of carbohydrate in a person's diet. Paige concludes that the patient community is more innovative and open to alternatives and is willing to accept the advice of a *crowd* of diabetics rather than a *crowd* of people she does not identify with.[4]

People participating in the TuDiabetes forum conversations regularly question the advice of medical providers as well. Here, the wisdom of the crowd comes through in the various responses a person gets to a question she asks. For example, the following responses were posted to answer one individual's question:

1. Sounds like my story. My doc put me on insulin, but still said it was type 2. After seeing the endo it was clear that it had been type 1 all along. Using insulin is a bit jarring at first, but actually you can eat more things you love if you count your carbs and take enough insulin to cover what you eat. You'll feel better too, and be less emotional/angry.
2. Find a new doctor, quickly. You need the blood work done. Your doctor should have done something for this. I have found with me it takes 3 weeks minimum for meds to kick in and bring my BG levels down and you are way past that.

Another discussion thread expresses similar concerns about the medical advice a community member is receiving. The person asks the crowd, "What do you guys think about my doctor? Is this pretty normal in your experience? I guess I expected to get a ton of help from my doctor and was surprised by her lack of concern." This post received swift and furious feedback, with members using words such as "blasé" and "disinterested" to describe doctors who are seen as not wanting "informed, questioning patients who want to take control of their treatment" and who "challenge their authority." By the end of the evening, eight people had replied with comments that registered obvious disgust, such as, "Sounds like you need a new doctor," "Get a new or another doctor. I don't know how the hell she knows her other patients are

---

3. Readers may remember Paige's tendency to evaluate differing pieces of advice from the previous chapter.

4. The diabetic medical community has become more accepting of low carbohydrate diets. Most research with these diets has focused on type 2 and gestational diabetes.

'non-compliant' since she apparently doesn't give them any directions to comply WITH. Jeez."[5]

Moving Expertise in Liminal Spaces

What is particularly interesting in these attributions of expertise is that a
person inhabits more than one patient subjectivity. Of course, both health
care providers and patients are constrained by the practices of institutional
structures in ways that resist such plasticity. These structures place patients in
opposition to medical providers, a point made clear in Parsons's (1951) con-
jectures of the sick role. Diabetics are also constrained by cultural norms of
patienthood. A patient is someone who is cared for and has an identity that is
constructed, at least partially, through the person's relationship with medicine
(Herzlich & Pierret, 1987, p. 146).

Patients still often fit into one of Anzaldúa's (1983, pp. 252–53) "little cub-
byholes" of binary subjectivities for health professionals as well. Clearly, there
is a great deal of diversity in how patients are perceived within the medical
community, but the website texts examined for this project and the interviews
with diabetes care providers suggest that a predominant view of patients with
diabetes continues to rely on traditional, static binary categories that cannot
account for rhetorical plasticity.

Most of the providers interviewed interacted with people with type 2 who
were referred to them by a doctor, and as Kathy, one of the pharmacists, noted,
"most of my referrals are uncontrolled or never been through DSME [disease
self management education] or is a new diagnosis." Other providers used
binary distinctions such as type 1 or type 2 to define their patient population
(table 5). As the table shows, there is variation in the responses, but there is
also a commonality of relying on numbers for definition as well as diabetes
type (1 or 2) and details about medication, age, and weight.

Nonprofit and corporate websites devoted to people with diabetes and
products for diabetes treatment reflect such binary categories as well. Here
these categories often fall in line with the organization's mission and audience.
Historically the ADA was more closely focused on people with type 2 and the
Juvenile Diabetes Research Foundation (JDRF) was positioned as its counter-
part for people with type 1. But today the ADA positions itself as a resource for

---

5. These examples first appeared in the author's 2011 article "Warp and Weft: Weaving the
Discussion Threads of an Online Community." *Journal of Technical Writing and Communication*, 41(1), 5–31.

TABLE 5. Characterizations of Patient Populations by Providers

PROVIDER PSEUDONYM	PROVIDER TYPE	CHARACTERIZATION OF PATIENT POPULATION
Greta	CDE	Almost exclusively, because 90–95 percent of the people who have diabetes really have type 2. It's more likely to be the older person, who is set in their ways, set in their eating habits.
Kathy	Pharmacist	Seventy-five percent of my patients are obese. Yeah . . . obese. Twenty-five percent, like maybe there's maybe 1 percent, less than 1 percent are at a healthy weight, and then the other 24 percent were overweight. But 75 percent of them are obese. By BMI guidelines of, you know, 25–29.9 being overweight. And anything 30 and above being obese. I have not had one type 1 patient yet. Of the patients enrolled in my program, 100 percent are type 2. And I'd say definitely less than 50 percent are on insulin. Most of them are on oral medications.
Amy and Scott	Pharmacists	Usually [type] 2—about 95 percent. Maybe we've had one type 1.
Susan	Dietician	I would say it's probably more type 2s although there are some insulin-dependent type 2s in the group. So there's patients that have type 2 who are on insulin, but I'd say the majority of the patients are type 2 diabetics.
Dr. Jackson	Primary care doctor	Type 1s, usually [on a] pump, but some on multiple injections.
Ken	Diabetes support group leader	[I] would say about half the people that come are generally newly diagnosed type 1 diabetics who are trying to make connections, figuring out, you know, everything that's happened to them, drawing on the experience of other diabetics. The other half are mostly type 2s but include a number of type 1s who are longer-term diabetics. And most of the people who come are adults, and I'd say the preponderance of people are age 40 and up.

people with all types of diabetes. As such, they include the different versions of the disease as part of their main website navigation. The main links on the "Diabetes Basics" web page include the following:

- type 1,
- type 2, and
- gestational diabetes.

Novo Nordisk, an insulin manufacturer, highlights information for type 1 patients, such as detailed information on insulin pens—including what the pens look like, the differences between various types of pens, why people may prefer them over insulin syringes, and the fact that some of the pens with thinner needles may hurt less than traditional syringes. Merck, a pharmaceutical company, manufactures oral medications for type 2 patients. Therefore, the company's website focuses on type 2. One resource available on the website, for example, is the workbook *Living Well with Diabetes,* which is published through a joint effort between Merck, the ADA, and StayWell. In the opening of the e-book, diabetes is defined as follows:

> Anyone can develop diabetes. It can affect people of all ages and backgrounds. But there are some common risk factors for diabetes. These include:
>
> - Family history of diabetes
> - Lack of physical activity
> - Being overweight
> - Being over age 45
> - Being African-American, Native American, Latino, Asian-American, Asian, Indian, or Pacific Islander
> - History of gestational diabetes (StayWell, 2015, p. 4)

These risk factors are all related to type 2 diabetes.

As with the binary sense of identity encouraged by a narrative of progress embedded in the provider texts examined in chapter 1, such divisions are not only pragmatic or economic. They also indicate a worldview in which patients are seen as one thing or another—novice or expert, type 1 or type 2, and controlled or uncontrolled. These identities of one or the other are linked to a singular view of the patient because in defining what a patient is, these texts also define what a patient is not. And while such classification seems a simple task, the work of classifying diabetes, like that of classifying tuberculosis that Bowker and Star (1999) describe, is complex. People with latent autoimmune diabetes in adults (LADA), which is similar to type 1 in that the person needs to inject insulin, often get misdiagnosed as having type 2 diabetes because they acquire the disease as adults rather than as children. The term *prediabetes* presents a similar classification complexity. It was first used to denote abnormalities of pregnancy or a strong family history of type 2 diabetes, but in 1980, the World Health Organization (WHO) discarded the term largely because of the fear that people with borderline blood sugar levels that did not progress to diabetes would unnecessarily worry. In 2005, however, the ADA reintroduced the term to refer to impaired glucose tolerance (IGT) and impaired fasting glucose (IFG) but not other risk factors for diabetes, such as obesity (Grundy, 2012). The classification systems structured by these organizations leave little room for ambiguity to "leave certain terms open for multiple definitions across social worlds" (Bowker & Star, 1999, p. 324). Such explanations are also problematic because of the "fluid, dynamic, and multiple" (Phillips, 2006, p. 310) nature of subjectivity that occurs because of articulations of expertise not only with multiple forms of knowledge but with multiple forms of expertise and multiple audiences.[6]

Enacting Multiple Patient Subjectivities

An unusual way multiple patient subjectivities surface online is through hijacking discussion forum threads. These threads are started by one person but hijacked by another. This action highlights the heterogeneity of the community and the discord that can underlie such communities, which we often ignore, but it also becomes an avenue for building expertise. In one such hijacked discussion thread, the original author of the thread starts out with a general cry for help: "I'm trying to take a deep breath here through the hiccups and tears." As the person continues to write, it becomes obvious that they have knowledge of their disease:

> I put i[t] [a blood glucose testing meter] in a cupboard and stayed in denial
> for months, despite some symptoms I knew belonged in the diabetes realm.
> I checked it yesterday with a visiting cousin, and it was 410. Called the after
> hour nurse who said I needed to go to the ER. 6 units of insulin later my
> numbers went up. 6 more units later, lots of blood work, I left at 2am, came
> home and fell into bed exhausted, waking up at 9:15 am to a fasting of 267.

And yet, the person does not identify as an expert until her thread is hijacked by someone else. Here is the hijacking post:

> Hi, just newly diagnosed here on 11/24/2009. I acquired my diabetes because
> of 2 different medications I took last year, both of which have the 'side effect'
> of causing diabetes in *rare* cases. Well, I just happen to be one of those
> *rare* cases. For me, diabetes IS a prison. I am stuck babysitting this horrible
> disease. It ruined my life and impacted the lives of those around me. It is a
> prison and I am its inmate. Sure, if I am good (i.e. keep blood sugars under
> tight control), I can get out for a moment (i.e. eat something I shouldn't), but

---

6. In describing discourse as an event that comes out of a set of practices and relations rather than a pre-existing reality outside of discourse, Foucault (1994) discusses subjectivity as a plural concept embedded in the subject's positions to various domains or objects and the information networks within which the speaker (in Foucault's case this referred to nineteenth-century doctors) operates.

have to return to it to finish my life sentence. I am not on any meds whereas you at least have the opportunity to more precisely control yours. Which CAN be done [. . .].

The hijacker begins with a typical opening for a newcomer to the community: "Hi, just newly diagnosed here on 11/24/2009." Most of the newcomers to the TuDiabetes community tend to post their diagnosis stories very soon after diagnosis, but when they do so they start their own discussion thread. Here, the person hijacks someone else's thread. Interestingly, one result of the action is that the original poster is afforded an opportunity to come back to the conversation as an expert. The original author of the thread responds to a post about what the hijacker has been eating:

> I'm not sure I understand? If you are eating 60-sometimes 250g of carbs per meal, what is there you cannot eat? What are you throwing out? I could eat an entire bowl of pasta with a limit of 250g? never mind soups and bread. I'm being honest here . . . I'm not here to judge anyone, just try to figure out as much as I can. It's not for me to judge if someone is drinking pop, or eating donuts. Anyhow, I'm already fat, and shots don't have any part in that. Plain, old-fashioned food did. Mind you I've been consistently losing since diagnosis the first week of January 2010. I eat as few carbs as I can, while my readings have been coming and staying down. I am learning my body, what I can tolerate. It sounds like you are too. I don't think I'd have good numbers if I personally ate cereal, milk, and a banana. I have to stick to more protein, veggies (which I gather you detest), and 10g of carbs or less per snack. I find it's not that hard to keep to that low carb idea when I eat proper portions. Likely it's what I should have been having all along. A single rye krisp cracker, with 2oz of lowfat cheese, truly does take an afternoon hunger pain away [. . .].

Similarly, not long after, the hijacker, who seems to be posting here as a new, uninformed member, starts dispensing advice:

1. 1st thing I would suggest is that you ask for Lantus. This can help even out blood sugars without bouncing too high or low once you get everything adjusted.
2. For me (NIDDM), diet and exercise alone—no meds. My last A1C was 5.8 One before that was 5.7. And at time of diagnosis, it was 6.8. I got everything down in a matter of 6 weeks roughly, all without any meds or formal diabetes education. [. . .]

These posts, like more traditional versions of illness stories, are public representations of individual identity. Here, by taking over the narrator position of the discussion thread, the hijacker assumes the identity as narrator of the tale and, in turn, gains narrative authority, an authority not dissimilar to the narrative competence addressed in chapter 2.

The movement back and forth between expert and novice positions in the discussion illustrates that people with diabetes, like health care professionals, enact several subject positions.[7] Still, the person with diabetes working in the spaces of online spaces and group appointments moves back and forth between technical subject-matter experts (medical providers) and less specialized audiences (families, friends and people newly diagnosed with diabetes).[8] But even this characterization is not quite adequate to describe the subjectivities of people with diabetes. A quotation from Tom helps explain the difference. In this excerpt, Tom, who sounded so expert in his opening comments, describes his interactions in a group appointment setting:

> I guess I am still somewhat timid to answer a lot of questions in the group setting. I do consider myself a rookie of the disease in that I haven't had it ten, fifteen, twenty years like some of the other folks in the room. I'm somewhat reserved in offering a lot. Whereas I understand more of the medical aspect, I'm still more new to the self-management. Some of the individual meetings, I certainly feel like I have to participate more because it's my appointment—so I need to ask a lot more questions and be more engaged and involved. With those support groups, I can take more of a passive role and just soak things in, and maybe offer things if I feel like I have a good idea. But just soak it all in. With those one-on-one meetings, I have to meet him halfway and be real forthcoming with answers and proactive questions.

Tom sees himself at once as a rookie in terms of lived experience because he has not been living with diabetes but a few years and yet as an expert of

---

7. Grounding much of his own theoretical stance in Mol's (2002) ideas about multiple ontologies, Graham (2009) has addressed the multisubjectivity of medical providers, stating that the "practices of health care professionals replicate both the structuralist accounts of ideological interpellation and the poststructuralist theories of multivocal subjectivity" (p. 378).

8. Building on Slack et al.'s (1993) theorization of the subjectivity of marginalized technical writers, Jeyaraj (2004) looks at technical authorship through the lens of critical theories about authorship, liminality, and colonization to try to better understand the marginalization of technical writers in their workplaces. He argues that defining technical writers as liminal subjects (by virtue of their rhetorical knowledge and skills) helps to shift this subjectivity and that liminal states are in fact agential because they have "the potential to change the current functioning of discourse" (p. 15).

the medical aspects of the disease because of his work experience, which is in a scientific laboratory. Tom not only shifts from a subjectivity of novice to expert or expert to novice, he sees himself as both at the same time. In other words, unlike technical writers who maneuver between two worlds, that of subject-matter experts and audiences/users, people with diabetes inhabit multiple subjectivities at the same time and walk in two worlds simultaneously. Norm, who had been diabetic for more than thirty years, similarly noted,

> I would not consider myself an expert, because I still don't know it all. I'm a semi-expert. I think I know what to do and how to do it fairly well, and I have improved at it considerably over when I started it. But I still have amazements.

These shifts are often apparent in online patient communities when someone begins a new type of therapy, such as moving from insulin injections to an insulin pump, or when a new life event occurs, such as when a woman with diabetes becomes pregnant. What becomes clear is that this movement between subjectivities of expertise and novice is anything but linear. If Norm, who has so many years of lived experience with the disease, can see himself as merely semi-expert, how could a narrative of linear progression be accurate?

ATTRIBUTED INTERACTIONAL EXPERTISE AND FLUID SUBJECTIVITIES

Unlike the journey of the Conversation Maps, people with diabetes do not experience a linear, one-way journey toward disease expertise. And yet, the experience people with diabetes have in the health care system tends to focus on two moments in time that stress such linearity. The first is that of the time of diagnosis, a fact made apparent in Medicare's policy for diabetes education. Medicare Part B covers 10 hours of *initial* diabetes self-management training to teach patients to cope with and manage their diabetes. As the pharmacists I spoke with noted, another time such education is put into place is when a doctor defines a patient as uncontrolled and refers the patient to an educational appointment.

The subjectivities people with diabetes embody are complex and multiple, but the ability to see oneself as at once an expert patient and a novice belies representations of people with diabetes that get created for them. Liminal spaces of chronic illness, on the other hand, are generative for such subjectivities or positions in relation to knowledge (i.e., expertise). In online communities and group appointments, diabetics do not just shift from one subjectivity to another. They are in fact *at once* teacher and student, expert and novice. The opening quotation of this chapter invokes a notion of subjects as multiple in a similar way. The *mestiza* rhetoric performed by Anzaldúa in the quotation is discourse that comes from a specific, complex cultural background, but it also more generally recognizes a kind of internal multiplicity and multiple subjectivities. As such, it creates tension with existing concepts of patient agency—a view that reinforces the concept of subjects as single and static entities—and subjectivity as a rhetorical form that "exists only in its continual and aesthetic creation, in its indefinite becoming" (Vivian, 2000, p. 304).[9]

This becoming and re-becoming in the form of multiple subjectivities is an important way that people with diabetes enact agency and expertise, but it is also important to note that even if not fixed, subjects are still situated.[10] Feminist scholarship has used the concept of positionality or situatedness to delineate how one's position influences the production of knowledge (Haraway, 1992). As Wolf (1996) puts it: "This approach goes beyond . . . and encourages us to think in terms of multiple perspectives and mobile subjectivities, of forging collaborations and alliances and juxtaposing different viewpoints. (pp. 14–15).[11] Positionality, in other words, is relational.

Because people with diabetes perform expertise through subjective matter knowledge (with episteme, techne, and bodily knowledge) and expertise through attribution, Hartelius's (2011) bounded categories of expertise are also problematic in terms of their ability to describe the relationship between subjectivities, agency, and expertise. People with diabetes occupy a number of subject positions and switch among them depending on the needs of a situation, and they often occupy more than one subject position at a time. Sometimes they demonstrate expertise through subject matter knowledge. At other times this expertise is attributed. In many ways the expert patient subjectivities diabetics inhabit make me think of the Four Corners Monument

---

9. Deleuze and Guattari (1987) also speak of subjectivity in terms of becoming. Their approach to subjectivity is not easily summarized, but we can take away that, for them, the self is "merely a collection of infinite and random impulses and flows" (Mansfield, 2000, p. 136), or what they refer to as lines of flight and machinic assemblages. Their metaphor of the rhizome challenges traditional Western thought that works to produce a "single authoritative and stable structure" (Mansfield, 2000, p. 143) from mobile, multiple relationships. In the case of the rhizome, the stable structure is the tree. The rhizome is in an eternal state of becoming, not working toward expressing an innate nature.

10. When Lucien Goldmann, a respondent to both Foucault's paper "What Is an Author?" and Derrida's paper "Structure, Sign, Play in the Discourse of the Human Sciences," asked both men "where is the subject?" both replied that they did not reject the subject. Rather, the subject has to be situated (Mansfield, 2000).

11. See also Alcoff, 1988.

where Arizona, Colorado, New Mexico, and Utah meet in the southwest of the United States. A visitor here can stand with one foot in Arizona and Utah and move to straddling Arizona and Colorado in a second.

The articulation of such subjectivities as multiple and fluid, unattached to assumptions about progress, problematizes an evolutionary view of moving from novice to expert patient. And because diabetics do not have one foot staunchly planted in the world of lived experience, the potential for multiple articulations is needed. Paraphrasing Hall (1985), Slack et al. (1993) point out the following about articulations: "Each identity [in a social formation] is actually a particular connection of elements that, like a string of connotations, works to forge an identity that can and does change" (p. 26). As such, these different articulations can "empower different possibilities and practices" (Slack, 1989, p. 331). For people with diabetes, these possibilities include perennial movement in subjectivity. Therefore, other models of expertise of subjectivity should be drawn upon.

If the subject is shifting and unstable, as Biesecker (1989) pointed out, the rhetorical event of shifting may be seen as an incident that "produces and reproduces the identities of subjects and constructs and reconstructs linkages [articulations] between them" (p. 126). Similar manifestations of subjectivity can be found in the contemporary literature of technical communication studies.[12] In the post-Information Age, knowledge work in hybrid spaces is characterized by continual movement and oscillation (Mol & Law, 2004)—of people, networks, places, and information. Graham (2009), for example, argues that individuals can occupy any number of subject positions and willfully switch among them, given the demands of the situation. Jeyaraj (2004) talks about this movement in terms of the relationship between the technical writer and subject matter expert.[13] Given the emphasis on collaborative work in technical communication workplaces, contributory expertise has been taken up as a useful way to discuss expertise (Henry, 1998). Spinuzzi (2008) introduced

---

12. Much of this work builds from the foundational text by Slack et al. (1993). Drawing on Foucault's work in the essay "What Is an Author?" they write that authorship is a way to valorize certain discourses over others and empower certain individuals while the contributions of other individuals remain invisible (Slack et al., 1993, p. 13). This statement has had a significant impact on research in technical communication, influencing work such as Winsor's extensive research into the work of engineers and technicians (1999, 2000, 2001, 2003, and 2006). Because technical discourse is not one of those discourses that is considered authored, technical communicators had been viewed as transmitters or translators of meaning. Slack et al. (1993) offered a solution to this conundrum through a third view, that of articulation (Deleuze & Guattari, 1981; Gramsci, 1971; Grossberg, 1987 and 1989; Hall, 1985, 1986, and 1996; and Laclau, 1977).

13. Historically, Jeyaraj (2004) reminds us, technical writers have been marginalized by subject matter experts (e.g., Grove, Lundgren, & Hays, 1992; Henry, 1994; Walkowski, 1991).

a similar concept in his book *Network* where he contrasted competence and expertise. Competence in actor-network theory, he explains, is "a property of the assemblage of humans and nonhumans" (p. 191) and competency emerges from the assemblage of human and nonhuman actors. Scholars in medical rhetoric and technical communication have paid less attention to what Collins (2004) sees as a midrange expert on the expertise continuums, interactional experts. If subjectivities of expertise are relational, such an interactional approach to expertise works with ideas of liminal subjectivity and relational agency, even though Collins and Evans (2007) offer what they call a realist approach rather than relational one. In their 2007 text, Collins and Evans use the metaphor of a five-step ladder to discuss expertise. This image, of course, is unfortunately similar to the ladder motif in some of the diabetes patient education material I have discussed. If we see expertise as existing on a spectrum, as Collins (2004) also indicates, however, we can draw less on its definition as a way to classify something on a point between two opposite poles, which suggests stability over time, and more on the idea that within a spectrum a subjectivity can vary infinitely within a continuum.[14]

In theorizing the idea of expertise in general and interactional expertise more specifically, Collins (2004) makes the distinction between a contributory expert—one who learns to make contributions to the field—and interactional experts—"Someone who can talk competently about aspects of a field . . . but only learns about the field from talking with people who have acquired contributory expertise" (Selinger & Mix, 2006, p. 303). The interactional expert has tacit knowledge but is not a direct practitioner in the field.[15] In other words, interactional expertise "is expertise in the *language* of a specialism in the absence of expertise in its *practice*" (Collins & Evans, 2007, p. 28). This interactional expertise is, therefore, useful for re-articulating patient identities with professional identities. Epstein (2000) applies such a view to the success of early AIDS activists, who used their technical expertise, or, in this case their expertise about the lived experience of the disease, and communication expertise to transform treatment practices. These experts try to affect practice through persuasion and language to bring about "changes in the epistemological practice of science" (Epstein, 2000, p. 16). Selinger and Mix (2006) go on

14. My use of the word *spectrum* should not be confused with many contemporary uses of the word *spectrum* in medicine, such as that of Autism Spectrum Disorder, in which the individual maintains a particular identity and the spectrum just refers to a cluster of similar symptoms that are grouped together.

15. Fountain (2014), on the other hand, argues that "communicative expertise, or the expertise involved in communication," and "technical expertise, or the specialized knowledge that professionals use in technical domains" (pp. 1–2), are not so easy to separate from each other.

to say that the activists' value as interactional experts "lies precisely in their ability to 'interact' with contributory experts in a way that provides the latter with a new understanding of how to best contribute to the advancement of medical science" (p. 306).

The interactional expertise witnessed in group sessions and online patient spaces is both immersive and relational. These interactions are immersive experiences—a form of experience Collins and Evans (2007) state is required to obtain specialized expertise—simply by the fact that multiple people with the experience of diabetes are participating in expertise acquisition at the same time. They are relational by virtue of their dependence on language, much as attributed expertise can be. Whereas attributed expertise relies on an audience that expertise is performed to, however, interactional expertise relies on a mutual communicative act. In these interactions people with diabetes can be seen as catalysts for others' expertise. In group appointments, providers perceived such interactions occurring. For example, a pharmacist said,

> In the group classes people are more willing to get more involved and ask questions—maybe because they feel more comfortable with other diabetics there versus maybe more on the spot. I don't know what it is, but in my brief experience it seems like there's more communication back and forth. There's more interaction. They kind of play off each other. One will ask a question, another will ask a related question, and they'll kind of go from there. . . . They can learn from each other though, like you were saying. Maybe they retain some of it more or actually use some of the knowledge a little bit better if someone who actually has it has done it—if they say it versus one of us, just sitting there lecturing people.

In a group visit that I observed for recruitment purposes, one individual talked about struggling to manage her blood sugar. Rather than jumping in as the expert and dispensing advice, the doctor asked the other participants what advice they had for the young woman. The other patients immediately took on the identity of expert and provided many different suggestions for what had worked for them despite the fact that they were taking part in a group medical appointment because the doctor identified them as novices (i.e., patients that needed education in order to better manage their blood sugar levels). This quick renegotiation of subjectivity is apparent in the conversations with diabetics about expertise as well. In these conversations people with diabetes can move into the role of expert, but in doing so they cross an invisible dotted line and in many ways they enter a liminal state (Turner, 1967 and 1974). They are not passive, uninformed patients. They are not medical experts who have gone to medical school, completed a residency, and set up a practice. Their position is much more fluid, and as my interviews show, this dotted line gets crossed time and time again as the "micro" exigence of practicing diabetes changes.

The shift in subject positions of people with diabetes is somewhat similar to what Phillips (2006) calls rhetorical maneuvers: "*a calculated action determined by the multiplicity of possible subjectivities*" (p. 321; emphasis in original). He notes the importance of articulation in this process, but states that a subject position gains validity "from the multiplicity of subject forms and the disruptive potential inherent in articulating an inappropriate subjectivity" (p. 321). He relates it to the classical notion of catachresis, the improper use of a word or stretching of a metaphor, which contemporary scholars (see Spivak, 1993 and Butler, 1993) have used to talk about people who are "erased from a form of discourse" (Phillips, 2006, p. 316). The rhetorical maneuver involves importing a name from another discourse. This name is somehow inappropriate for the current discourse formation and as such "challenges the contours of the subject position and the proper subject form it encourages." (Phillips, 2006, p. 316). Phillips uses an example to illustrate:

> After class a student approaches me and states, "I've missed some work in the last week and would like to make it up." Now, at this point, the regular rules of discourse are in place—I am in the superordinate position and the student in a subordinate one. We are both speaking from established positions within a larger formation of discourse and, up to this point, speaking within the appropriate forms as "student" and "professor." However, the student continues, "I think my girlfriend is pregnant and we've both been really upset." (p. 317)

Phillips argues that in this example, the student tries to disrupt the regular patterns of both his and his professor's subject positions by introducing an inappropriate subject position into this particular discursive formation—his future status as a father. People with diabetes do not seek to disrupt or resist through rhetorical maneuvers, however. Instead, rhetorical plasticity enables alternate articulations for more appropriate subject position in the set of relations the person is operating within. Elliott offers an example in his tendency to move back and forth in terms of identity as expert. Elliott was part of a focus group in which he was the member who had lived with diabetes the longest time. Interestingly, this participant responded immediately to my questions, establishing himself as a pack leader, so to speak. The group itself also seemed to defer to his expertise by giving him the floor first as the participants responded to questions and, in fact, arranged all their responses in order of who had been a member of the community the longest: Veteran members spoke first and the newer members followed.

Elliott established his expertise by telling the group the length of time he had been a member of the community and the length of time he had been living with diabetes.

> ELLIOTT: I tell you, when I came on there were about, there were about 5,000 participants when I came on, so Manny would probably be able to tell you better when that was. Well, for me, and I've been diabetic, I'm a type 1, and I have been for 35 years and I define good control as anything that is on a routine basis less than 100 and I define out of control anything greater than 200. So, in that 100 to 200 spread, that's where the line changes for me somewhere in there . . . depending on the time of day.

In the following excerpt, Elliott downplays his expertise as a patient in his insistence on the importance of listening to the advice of medical professionals. The second excerpt similarly discusses his trepidation about giving advice to people in the online social networking community to which he belongs.

> ELLIOTT: Whenever I give advice I always start with "listen to your doctor" and I will sometimes say, "you know, this is what I have done, however, I do suggest you listen to your doctor." One of the things I think is probably off limits is when folks knowingly and persistently contradict medical professionals in a patient's life. I try to be careful of the advice I give, not that I'm uncomfortable giving it, it's just that I don't want to say, you know, what works for me necessarily worked for other folks. And I don't want to give somebody the wrong advice. So I probably will give less advice than perhaps others, but the advice I give I'm comfortable giving. I've only gotten in trouble once.

As the interview continued, however, Elliott moved back to a role as expert as he describes his role within the online community.

> ELLIOTT: Well I am a user, contributor. I am a person who reads it [the website] just about every day. I'm a person who comments probably once every two weeks, and I'm a person who has sole responsibility for my own care. I do not believe doctors [. . .]. I don't really think that doctors or anybody else really has all the information to make a proper decision about me. So I treat them as a good source of advice, but I don't recall ever doing something a doctor said just because they said it.

Elliott's comment about treating the information doctors give him as advice rather than objective truth indicates that he, similar to Paige, is evaluating the doctors' expertise. As such, he enacts expertise himself. Sara also quickly runs through these roles in a single response to my question about her role in the online community she is a member of:

> SARA: I'm still trying to figure out what my role with TuDiabetes is going to be. I have commented on people who I've had some more experiences with just to offer support, and kind of like a shoulder to lean on at this point. Which is very similar to, strangely enough, with some of my students who are type 1 diabetics who are at this point in their lovely teenage years and aren't ready to focus on the disease and ready to deal with the reality of the disease. With my doctors, [my] primary and I actually have a running joke going. She won't touch anything related to my diabetes because her comment is, "you know way more than I do about it because you've dealt with it as long as you have." If I need to go in and say, "look, I'm having issues with numbers during this time frame, can you look up and double check to make sure my logic and reasoning is right?" She doesn't have a problem doing that and in fact encouraged me to go and find a different endocrinologist because the endocrinologist I was working with at the time, things just weren't clicking and I wasn't getting the help and support that I needed to help get things back in control. I would say I probably am the lead on the health care team going, "look, this is what I want—I want to get my A1C to the 6 to 6.5 range." Particularly since I'm actually looking at going back to school full time for 27 months and I know what that means to my body and that I need to get things back on track and get things back and going forward, especially since I do want to go on and do something with endocrinology.

As a new member to the online networking community, Sara does not feel expert enough to offer advice to others, but she does feel expert enough to control her own medical treatment with her doctor. She also feels expert enough in her role as a high school teacher in relation to her students with type 1 diabetes.

Segal (2005) notes that the "competence gap" (p. 146) between patients and physicians has been a topic of discussion for well over fifty years and that "a rhetorical view of advice and adherence suggests the usefulness of a negotiation of expertise" (Segal, 2005, p. 147). In this statement, the author specifically addresses this negotiation as one between providers and patients. The provider texts discussed in this chapter support this view: My provider participants and texts offer a narrative of patients that show them as people who need to become experts, and in this narrative the providers are positioned to facilitate a transfer of knowledge to patients to close this gap. People with diabetes, however, negotiate their roles as experts in relation to one another in a way that does not correspond with this narrative. Rather than a negotiation between the self and a provider, it is one between knowledge, other patients' experiences, and their own bodily experiences. Such negotiations are less visible in one-on-one appointments between providers and patients. In collaborative group educational settings, however, these broader negotiations come to light. By negotiating and renegotiating their positions within the discursive situation, diabetics challenge the long-held assumptions about patient agency that rely on articulations to autonomy. These alternating performances of subjectivity as expert and nonexpert and all the spaces in between show us how the so-called competence gap is actually not a gap at all. Rather, it is but one space among many within the perpetual state of liminality in which agency is enacted in diabetes, a state in which roles are not static, immobile subjectivities but rather temporary articulations and performances.

CHAPTER 5

Mimesis and Identification

The Patient as Professional

> First, the instinct of imitation is implanted in man from childhood, one dif-
> ference between him and other animals being that he is the most imitative of
> living creatures, and through imitation learns his earliest lessons.
>
> —Aristotle, *Poetics*

PEOPLE WITH diabetes have traditionally been viewed as expert patients because diabetics (rather than medical professionals) are experts in the area of the lived experience of their disease. As such, concepts like identification and peer mentoring have been increasingly looked at as valuable tools in patient education for people with diabetes. If diabetes is healthwork, however, people with diabetes also need to have a professional identity that shifts their status from that of a patient outside the health system to a professional member of the medical neighborhood. But how does a patient gain access to such an identity? In applying Burke's (1950) concept of identification and Perelman and Olbrechts's (1969) adherence theory to a study of compliance, Segal (1994) argues that the asymmetry inherent in the doctor-patient relationship excludes the possibility of identification. However, articulations in collective, liminal spaces do in fact make this type of identification possible. One such articulation is between mimesis—imitating the words or actions of another—and enactments of professional identities.

Given the negative connotations that mimesis has acquired throughout history, mimesis as performances of professionalism might seem counterintuitive in terms of generating positive change or agency.[1] Although Plato

---

1. Mimesis has a variety of meanings in classical rhetoric (McKeon, 1936; Corbett, 1971; Goodnight & Green, 2010). McKeon (1936) describes it as "a constant relation between something which is and something made like it: the likeness itself may be good or bad, real or

made more than 10 associations to mimesis in *The Republic* (Melberg, 1995), the one that has persisted is in Book 10, the definition that ranks imitation below truth. Even in a contemporary culture that values remix as a form of invention, we have misgivings about imitation. Take, for example, the negotiations between musicians Sam Smith and Tom Petty involving the similarity of the song "Stay With Me"—written by Sam Smith, James Napier, and William Phillips—to Tom Petty and Jeff Lynne's song "I Won't Back Down." Although the argument about the originality of Smith's song never became a lawsuit, according to Petty, Petty and Lynne ended up receiving songwriting credit (and therefore songwriting royalties) for what Petty refers to as a "musical accident" (Petty, 2015, para. 1).

Mimesis does, however, have another dimension that supports the recursive nature of agency in liminal spaces. Mimesis as repetition, Melberg (1995) explains, is "always the meeting-place of two opposing but connected ways of thinking, acting and making" (p. 1). Mimesis, in other words, shares liminal spaces' ability to bring together discourses of lived experience and clinical medical knowledge. Along with sharing characteristics of liminality, mimesis shares characteristics of agency as "inherently, protean, ambiguous, open to reversal" (Campbell, 2005, p. 2) through its own inherent nature as a movable concept. Being between—between art and reality, representation and truth, or science and lived experience—mimesis becomes a strategy for both providers and people with diabetes to use as a way to cultivate temporary agency through present-tense performances of discourse. Much as identity can be performed and leveraged in "small, momentary, and fleeting acts" in the exchanges on a museum blog (Grabill & Pigg, 2012, p. 101), through mimesis people with diabetes can perform professional identities but still retain the ability to shift back to the discourse of lived experience and the expert patient. The rest of this chapter outlines three specific agential articulations that mimesis enables. The first involves representations of patients and providers in reported speech, the discourse practice of restating or reenacting talk (of others or oneself) that occurred at another place (Hengst, Frame, Neuman-Stritzel, & Gannaway,

---

apparent" (pp. 6–7). Corbett (1971) cites the function of imitation as follows: "For it is that internalization of structures [accomplished through imitation] that unlocks our powers and sets us free to be creative, original, and ultimately effective" (p. 250). Crowley (1985) also understands imitation as an attempt "to perfect the presentation of an old theme through adding, changing, or omitting" rather than "slavish copying" (p. 24). Finally, Leff (1997) states, "*Imitatio* is not the mere repetition or mechanistic reproduction of something found in an existing text. It is a complex process that allows historical texts to serve as equipment for future rhetorical production" (p. 201). For more comprehensive histories of the term *mimesis*, see Eric Auerbach's 2003 work entitled *Mimesis*.

2005). The second and third demonstrations are those of people with diabetes mimicking scientific ethos as a way to construct a professional identity.

RE-STATING

In general, reported speech takes two forms: direct and indirect. Direct reported speech presents the original speaker's words as if they were quoted directly, such as in the following example from one of my participants with diabetes:

> TERRI: My blood sugar was 933. So, I ended up in the hospital. Just before I was released, they set me up with Dr. Jackson. They said, "We'll make an appointment for you to see Dr. Jackson tomorrow."

If Terri's statement had been indirect reported speech, she might have said, "They said that they'd make an appointment for tomorrow."

Whether direct or indirect, the term *reported speech* carries journalistic implications of accuracy and objectivity, but there is no guarantee that these utterances are accurate in terms of what was originally said (Tannen, 1989). For example, in Clark and Gerrig's (1990) study in which researchers asked participants to listen to two-sentence conversational exchanges then asked them to accurately quote the exchange they participated in, none of the 10 participants were able to do so in a total of 720 tries. Because reported speech does not function as an accurate representation of a statement that someone made in the past, a person makes choices about how a person, situation, or event is represented when they use this discursive strategy. As such, reported speech can be seen as a form of heteroglossia (Bakhtin, 1981) that has agential qualities.[2]

Although reported speech has been defined as a ubiquitous phenomenon (Vološinov, 1973), the majority of research presupposes a narrative discourse frame (Baynham, 1996). Research related to medical rhetoric has focused on the reported speech of medical professionals in relationship to their professional identities. Catherine Schryer and her co-researchers, in particular, have discussed reported speech as a boundary object between people in adjacent professional spheres, such as those of law and medicine (Schryer, Bell, Mian, Spafford, & Lingard, 2011), and its role in professional identity formation for

---

2. Bakhtin (1981) defined heteroglossia as the combining of different ways of viewing the world that gets expressed through language. The languages of these different worldviews do not "*exclude* each other, but rather intersect with each other in many different ways" (p. 291).

social work students and medical students (Schryer, Campbell, Spafford, & Lingard, 2006). Drawing on a set of data that includes interviews with medical students and students preparing to become social workers, the authors examine the linguistic strategies these groups used to present what the authors refer to as cited information of the patient in order to transform patient/client information into professional data relevant for their respective fields. The authors note that the process was particularly important because it also demonstrated how people new to the field learn communication strategies that help shape their professional identities and can be useful in uncovering similarities and differences in the professions that might help them to find common ground when working together. They also note that social work students were encouraged to quote directly and even recreate their conversations with their patient/clients, but medical students rarely ever quoted their patients and instead used indirect reported speech patterns.[3]

Other studies investigate the effects that recasting patients' speech in provider notes has on patient identity.[4] Finally, reported speech research has focused on looking at how the reported speech used by medical providers creates patient identities. Ravotas and Berkenkotter (1998) have found that the initial written assessment documents psychotherapists compose: (1) depict a patient's meanings and (2) construct a clinical case to support the psychotherapist's diagnosis of the patient. In their study of letters and reports exchanged between optometrists and ophthalmologists, for example, Spafford, et al. (2008) note that these health care providers seldom quoted their patients in an analysis of 35 optometry referral letters. And although the appearance of patient voices is not the norm in such letters, its inclusion appears to accomplish specific work: to persuade reader action, to question patient credibility, and to highlight patient agency.

The reported speech utterances of the providers interviewed for this project had functions similar to those reported by Spafford, et al. (2008)—persuading a patient and questioning a patient's credibility. In this case, however, persuasion is communicated through complying with medical authority, making agency problematic. As discussed in the second half of this chapter, however, opportunities for agency do emerge through the performances of reported speech.

---

3. Also see Schryer, Lingard, Spafford, and Garwood (2003); Schryer and Spoel, (2005); and Spafford, Schryer, Mian, and Lingard, (2006).

4. See Hak and de Boer (1996); Mishler (1984); Schryer et al. (2011); Spafford, Schryer, and Lingard (2008).

Persuading through Reported Speech

To persuade patients, providers most often used directives re-quoting in their own voices as voices of authority, such as in the following examples.

> SUSAN: So, keeping on a regular schedule is another issue. You know, many
> of them eat out; they don't time their meals very well; they eat when
> they're hungry. You know, they eat because of habit, not necessarily
> because of hunger, so some of it was just linking, you know? "You need
> to manage your diabetes better so that you don't have complications
> later."
>
> AMY: "We want you to check your blood sugar three times between now and
> next time." So the next time they come in we ask them, "how'd you do
> checking your blood sugar?"

The reported speech that providers used in talking about their interactions with patients positions them as authorities over their patients in two ways. The first is evident in their choice of reporting verbs. Writers use reporting verbs to evaluate the correctness of their sources and portray their sources as (1) presenting correct information with verbs such as *acknowledge* or *demonstrate*, (2) presenting false information using verbs such as *betray* or *disregard*, and (3) presenting no clear signal as to the writer's attitude about the source's credibility, using verbs such as *claim* or *propose* (Thompson & Ye, 1991). They also use reporting verbs to indicate how their source material fits into their own interpretation. Professionals use reporting verbs such as *report, argue,* or *describe* to suggest that a writer (or speaker) may represent reported information as

- true (acknowledge, point out, establish);
- false (fail, overlook, exaggerate, ignore);
- non-factive (giving no clear signal). (Hyland, 2000, p. 28)

Medical providers in this study use reporting verbs to indicate that they see themselves as objective sources of the information:

> DAISY: I said, "It helps to review and go back, because even when I go back
> and read some of this, it means something different to me a year later.
> So, I strongly encourage you to fit that somewhere in, like before you're
> going to go see your doctor, or right after you've gone to see your doctor.

Just review, and then you're more aware of questions to ask, or things they are saying might make better sense."

The advice that providers give through reported speech is unquestioningly seen as fact; therefore, there is no need to *propose* or *argue*. They simply need to *say*. Providers also positioned themselves as authorities in the use of directives phrased as imperative sentences, sentences used to give a command. While the subject of an imperative statement may be implied, that subject will always be *you*: *You* need to manage your diabetes better; just check *your* blood sugar every day. People who have authority over others use imperative sentences as a way of establishing this authority. In these examples, therefore, the providers see themselves as experts directing or persuading patients to do certain things. The patients are simply expected to comply or carry out this work. The following excerpt from Kathy's interview illustrates this assertion. In chapter 2, Kathy explained that she goes through the material in her class.

> Then, at the end, I will go around and take blood pressures one by one and weights. You know, blood pressure, weight, blood pressure, weight, blood pressure, weight. But before I do blood pressures and weights, I say, "Now you need to write a goal for the next time."

She continues:

> When I open my next class, I'm going to say, "You set a goal last week of, you know, [she offers the following as an example of a goal the patient might have set] eating breakfast at least every day. Did you meet that goal?" Or, "you said you're going to exercise twice a week for 30 minutes. Did you meet that goal?" So, we discuss that at the beginning of class. And then also blood pressures and weights at the end. If they say, "I want to lose weight," then I have to say to them, "Okay, you want to lose weight, but healthy weight loss is one or two pounds a week. We could write that, but how are you going to do that? Are you going to exercise more? Eat less?" So then what is one step I can make, so okay, "I'm going to watch my portion size," you know? How am I going to accomplish my goal [reading from the sheet]? Well, they could measure their food and write it down, keep a food log. What conditions have to exist to meet my goal? Sometimes that's making sure that they go to the grocery and make sure they have the right food in the house versus being stuck to go eat fast food or something like that. Am I dependent on someone else? Well, "do you do the grocery shopping?" Then, when it comes to this,

how likely [is it that] I am going to do it? If they write down a five, well, then we better start over because if it's five or less, chances are you're not going to do it [the scale is zero to 10]. "Don't write it down for *me* [emphasis in original], write it down for *you* [emphasis in original]."

The way Kathy talks about setting goals sounds like this task provides a source for agency for the patient, as noted in chapter 2. The patient is writing the goal on the handout the pharmacist provides, and Kathy emphasizes that the goal setting is for the patient rather than the provider. The handout itself, however, conflicts with the idea that the patient is in charge. The bottom of the handout has a place for the patient and provider to sign and then an area in which the provider assesses the patient's performance in meeting this goal. The final line for sign off is the provider's, not the patient's. The providers in my study seem to have a genuine interest in helping patients achieve this agency. Kathy, for instance, says writing is an important way to help empower her patients: "Now you need to write a goal for the next time." The handouts created by the pharmacy system that she is employed by, however, work against this interest and seem to embed both patient and provider in a compliance mindset, much like the documents Stone examined in 1997.

As such, questions about providers' own professional identity and agency emerge. These were not part of the original research question, but providers' use of reported speech in identity construction became apparent in the data. For some providers, reported speech patterns emphasized the structure and constraints of the hierarchal system of health care, a system that, despite efforts to change, still places value in dispensing advice and treatment orders. This value is evident in the directive language on both organizational websites and in the ADA's *Standards of Medical Care* document. For example, Joslin's website advises, "Learn as much about diabetes as possible. Most people don't know much at first, so this is not easy."[5] The text goes on to equate this learning process to taking a post-graduate course while feeling overwhelmed emotionally. Novo Nordisk offers advice about healthy eating using the word *want* (i.e., a person will want to eat in this manner). The use of the word *want* is not typical in all the directive texts examined from providers, but as it is used here, the emphasis is still on what the patient *should* do rather than what the patient *wants*. The directive language mimics the language in the *Standards of Medical Care* (ADA, 2016), as the following two quotations from the document show:

---

5. Copyright © 2016 by Joslin Diabetes Center. All rights reserved. Reprinted with permission from www.joslin.org.

1. "Aggressive interventions and vigilant follow-up should be pursued for those considered at very high risk (e.g., those with A1C > 6.0% [42 mmol/mol])." (p. S15)

2. "Widespread clinical testing of asymptomatic low-risk individuals is not currently recommended due to lack of approved therapeutic interventions. Higher-risk individuals may be tested, but only in the context of a clinical research setting. Individuals who test positive will be counseled about the risk of developing diabetes, diabetes symptoms, and DKA prevention." (p. S16)

As McCarthy (1991) illustrates in her essay about how influential the *Diagnostic and Statistical Manual of Mental Disorders* (DSM) is in shaping what a psychiatrist knows and communicates in her diagnostic work, the *Standards of Medical Care* influences how providers working in the area of diabetes care communicate. In mimicking the language of the guidelines, the providers' reported speech has a similar goal of establishing a professional identity by linguistically positioning the person with diabetes within the framework of science, medicine, and the delivery of health care. Reading from the instructional sheet Kathy gives patients, she says,

> How am I going to accomplish my goal [pointing to the text on the sheet]? Well, they could measure their food and write it down, keep a food log. What conditions have to exist to meet my goal [pointing to the text on the sheet]?

She follows the structure of the handout without deviating from it in her patient sessions, just as she did in describing the process of using the handout. Daisy followed a similar pattern as she began describing her process of using Conversation Maps. In the interview, Daisy walked around the map she had placed on the floor of the reception area of a doctor's office in which she held her group sessions. She explained,

> This idea actually started with a group of diabetes educators. It went a very circuitous route through [the] American Diabetes Association, an organization called Healthy Interactions, and they were really the guiding force at that point when they got ahold of it and said, "Yes, we can work with something that will stimulate conversation and stimulate give and take, instead of looking at the lecture idea of talking about diabetes." [. . .] So, when they do this, they have five maps. Each map has a facilitator's guide. "On the Road to Better Managing Your Diabetes" is the first one. They give you great detail of how to do the session, but then they leave it up to you as to what you do

and exactly what you say. But they give you tips along the way and things to say back to people, giving them encouragement, and making sure you're not shutting anybody down, and still learning what diabetes is, what the differences are between type 1 and type 2. . . . Okay. *So right here we start with* the definition [of diabetes]. *Medicines, up here.* Taking medicines. There used to be, like insulin. Then there was one oral medicine. Now we have six different classifications with maybe as many as six different medicines in each one of those classifications that you can take, so you and your doctor can work out which ones you need for what, because they target different things. Insulin is one of the medicines that when somebody is diagnosed and their blood sugar is really high, like over 300, then they put them on insulin right away. It doesn't mean they have to stay on it, necessarily. But it is a medicine that works, and getting that blood sugar down to a comfortable level is the aim. *We put it right there.* Most people are scared to death of needles. Oh, they think it's going to hurt like it's the longest needle and most painful injection they've ever had. . . . If you're newly diagnosed, you stand a very good chance of being able to do that. But if you've had diabetes for ten years or so, which many people have when they're first diagnosed, you aren't going to do it alone with diet and exercise; you're going to need some help. *Then, getting support.* Getting help from those who are important to you: family members. I always use some handouts here to remind people of their overall management plan. (emphases added)

Each time Daisy used one of the phrases emphasized in italics she would point to the Conversation Map, her guide as well as her patients' guide through the educational session. And though Daisy said that the Conversation Map program developers "leave it up to you as to what you do and exactly what you say," the journey motif embedded in the visuals and metaphors used in the maps encourages facilitators to follow this narrative of progress.

In her group educational appointments, Daisy would always stop the preplanned journey to answer questions, but she would also always come back to the template that the program developers provided. As such, there is a tension in terms of power and agency in her own performances of professional identity. On the other hand, Daisy in particular used a form of reported speech that intertwined clinical and lived experience that was agential in terms of resisting the narrative constructed for her. She intertwined tales of her sessions and patients with tales of exchanges she has had with people in her own family who have diabetes.

DAISY: My mother, when she was diagnosed with type 2 diabetes, she was into peanut butter. She'd eat about half a jar a day. I said, "Whoa, peanut butter is a good food, but not half a jar a day! So, Mom, what are we going to do here?" She solved it. This is what you want them to do, to do their own problem solving.

Daisy's use of reported speech was significantly different from other providers' use. This is likely due in part to personality differences: Daisy seemed to be a natural storyteller. Still, her storytelling use of reported speech might be related to her own expression of agency. I did not collect demographic data from my provider participants, but Daisy shared her background, history, and age. In her midseventies, she was the oldest provider interviewed. And even though she was tied to the text she was using, the Conversation Map, this form fit her own teaching style and in some ways freed her to be her own agent in terms of teaching her patients.

Questioning Patient Credibility

Providers also used reported speech as a way to question patients' credibility and conduct. In these utterances in particular, it was clear that as a framework of care, compliance has not lost power. One pharmacist's statement about a particular patient illustrates a perception of people with diabetes as being a noncompliant patient group: "Yes, because there's been a handful of patients— even the pharmacists have told me—with a difficult patient they've told me up front, 'They're not going to change anything, you know, so good luck.'" In this example, the reported phrase is actually reported twice: The pharmacists said it to the dietician, and the dietician said it to me during the interview. The language used paints a picture of a *problem patient,* someone who will not listen to advice or comply with directives given to them by medical professionals. Another example of this evaluative reported speech occurred near the end of the interview with Kathy.

I'm just amazed, especially with something like diabetes. It affects every part of your body and everything you do affects it, so I just think it's so important to learn everything there is about it. And it's kind of unfortunate that it takes so much time, but it's also important to devote that much time to it because it's so involved.

As the discussion moved to drawbacks to group appointments, Kathy added the following:

> I think that one of the drawbacks that people have when they get enrolled in this program is, "Oh, it's 10 hours. I don't have time for class; I don't even have time to exercise." You know what I mean?

In and of itself, this statement does not seem like a particularly negative evaluation of the patient. However, in the context of Kathy's previous statement, the characterization of a patient not making time for a disease that she sees as being so important to devote time to creates a negative evaluation of the patient profile she described. Other evaluative statements make this negative view apparent as well. In the following two excerpts, for example, the provider focuses on the areas still needing improvement as much as the areas in which the patient is doing well. The second excerpt, much more directive and direct, implies that the patient being spoken to in the reported speech is not taking care of his disease.

1. "They did well in these areas; they probably still need improvement in these areas."
2. "You need to manage your diabetes better so that you don't have complications later."

The view of patients as not complying or not willing to make an effort to engage in healthy behaviors is apparent in the evaluative statements that providers made about patients in reported speech, but none offered scenarios in which the patient was doing well or trying. Patients were always seen as resistant at best, an observation that can be extended to many classroom instructors, who are much more inclined to complain about students as problems—and about problem students—than to reflect positively on students who are doing really well in their courses.[6]

RE-STATING EXPERT PATIENTS AS PROFESSIONALS

Unlike medical professionals, patients typically do not have access to educational settings and professional organizations. Sometimes undergraduate and graduate students will shadow a professional to learn more about how that

---

6. The author acknowledges and thanks Wayne Hall for bringing this observation to her attention.

person does her job. But this is also not an option for people with the disease. They do not have the same access to write authoritative documents such as prescriptions or care guidelines either. People with diabetes do, however, find ways to create a professional identity for themselves through discourse and practices. To create these professional identities, diabetics rely on those things that set them apart rather than the things that link them together, invoking the second principle of identification Burke (1950) discusses, that of being "distinct substance" as well as "consubstantial with another" (p. 21).

Identifying with Health Care Professionals

Reported speech and hedging language used in reported speech are discursive indications of identifying with what has long been seen as distinct subjects—patients and doctors. Such language crosses terrain that may be less distinct and more slippery—an identity of expert patient and one of a healthworker. In the previous chapter, for example, Sara is described as a peer mentor (a type of expert patient). And yet, in the reported speech she uses in her advice on the effect of steroids on blood sugar levels ("Yours might be different, but this is what I tried and this is what worked."), Sara indicates that she is *more expert* than the person with diabetes she is addressing. Even though Sara knows another person's experience of the disease is likely to be different from hers, she uses an imperative statement (this is what works), indicating a command more than a choice. Nikki is another example of this fluid identity boundary. Although she says she "mentor[s] people from time to time and probably on things that are the everydays of this disease that aren't going to be in a text-book or your doctor may not necessarily know about it," she also aligns herself with medical professionals. In the same response, she gives examples of the kinds of questions she answers for people:

> You know, like, "I'm so stressed out, life is so stressful. Why are my num-bers so high?" You know? People will come to me with simple, everyday questions like that, or, you know, "How do I enjoy myself? My birthday's coming up, and how do I deal with food or how do I deal with food on the holiday," or, "I'm sick and why is my blood sugar high? I have a cold; why is it so high?" Things like that. Just the little, simple questions that some people might have, or concerns of day-to-day life. I tend to help people with that a lot.

Nikki aligns herself with medical experts by providing answers to "simple questions." She knows that most people with diabetes will see their doctor every few months, but between those visits are gaps of time in which hundreds of questions can come up, including dealing with changes in dietary patterns for holidays. Through her stance as a mentor, Nikki in some ways fills the function of the ask-a-nurse hotline some health care systems offer, hotlines staffed by nurses 24 hours a day to answer people's medical and health questions.

Nikki's identity as both peer mentor and professional creates an ambiguity—and ambiguity, as Burke (1945) notes, is a necessary and generative process in language. Burke (1945) illustrates beautifully with his example of molten rock. In this description, he suggests that once the mutation of presumed absolutes is allowed, everything is open to change and transformation. It is the ambiguity in language that allows us, in fact requires us, to interpret and re-interpret. Mimesis provides one mechanism for such rhetorical plasticity. It does not disable access to lived experience but enables simultaneous articulations to an expert patient identity and professional identity. It both signals and enables the identification Segal (1994) found lacking in patient-provider encounters. Despite the fact that when providers use reported speech it distances patients from such an identity, people with diabetes employ the strategy: They distance themselves from identities as expert patients and align with identities as professionals. These new identities are apparent in interactions with nondiabetics such as family members or a boss who thinks a person with type 1diabetes can cure their diabetes with diet and exercise. A frustrated member of the TuDiabetes online patient community posted the following about her boss, for example:

> He said I don't need to take insulin every time I eat something. He said having a low blood sugar is not an emergency and he will not allow me to take a break to eat or drink something. He said that it's not even a real disease and to leave my medical kit (my insulin and testing supplies) at home . . . that I'm just trying to make people feel sorry for me. He said you don't need to test your blood sugar multiple times a day or "shoot up" at work.

In being more expert than her boss, this person aligns herself with other experts in health care, trying to educate her boss about the disease and even echoing some health practicioners' frustration of patients looking things up online before coming in for an appointment: "I tried to explain to him that my type one diabetes is a very real life threatening disease and it is very necessary for me to test my BG and take my insulin. He said he looked up diabetes on 'Google' and I'm trying to make it worse than it really is."

Identifying with Scientific Research Professionals

People with diabetes also identify with scientific researchers through the use of hedging language in their reported speech. Hedging language has been identified as a characteristic of academic writing, particularly scientific writing, as Fahnestock (1986) pointed out almost thirty years ago in the article in which she investigates genres written for scientific audiences versus those written for nonscientific audiences. The language in the *Standards of Medical Care* (ADA, 2016b) often includes a level of certainty, but hedging language is evident as well. For example, the standards use the directive *should*: "All individuals with diabetes should receive individualized MNT [medical nutrition therapy], preferably provided by a registered dietitian who is knowledgeable and skilled in providing diabetes-specific MNT" (p. S25). At the same time, the document includes the use the more indefinite word *may*: "These devices [CGMs] may offer the opportunity to reduce severe hypoglycemia for those with a history of nocturnal hypoglycemia" (p. S40). The use of command words such as *should* and *cannot* contain a level of certainty (Fahnestock, 1986). They function linguistically in a similar way as news stories of scientific findings do, which drop the nuance of words like *suggest* and report findings as *proven*. In other words, when scientists talk to scientists, uncertainty is often retained in language. When scientific information is written for public audiences, it is more typical to see language that indicates certainty. Interestingly, in this study, when provider interviewees recast patient voices in relation to each other (rather than in relation to a medical professional), rather than phrasing this language as a directive, the providers used hedging language, a discursive move suggesting one expert talking to another. For example, using reported speech to characterize an exchange with a patient, a provider might say, "You should stick to your meal plan." If providers were reporting what one patient said to another, however, they would couch the more directive verb *should* in less directive language: "I think you should follow your meal plan."

People with diabetes use hedging language to a similar effect. Tom (a type 1) gives another example of the use of hedging language in a response to a question about his definition of control if another patient were telling him about his particular situation:

I *may say*, "You have relatively good control," whereas if I was looking at myself and had those same values, I would *maybe be* more motivated to make it better. I have a different idea of good control for myself than I would for a larger group of people. (emphasis added)

This type of language was apparent in the discourse of people with diabetes more generally as well. Consider the conversation about the definition of control from earlier chapters. Patrick's comment is a part of a discussion in chapter 1, and Mary's is part of an exchange in chapter 2:

> PATRICK: Yeah, I'm also a type 1 diabetic, late onset. I was diagnosed in 2008, so I'm still relatively new at this, but I define control *for me* [emphasis added] as sticking in the 140 range. Generally I run 105 and I rarely go over 200, once or twice a month. An A1C below 6.
>
> MARY: From a different perspective, *for me* [emphasis added] being in control means having an A1C that is as close to 6 as possible and being on no meds. But that's type 2.

Patrick and the other people with diabetes who were interviewed consistently used this phrase "for me." Whether used in conjunction with reported speech or by itself, the use of hedging language embraces the TuDiabetes community's policies and values. The community's editorial policy, for example, states,

> The contents of TuDiabetes is for informational purposes only and is not intended to be a substitute for professional medical advice, diagnosis, or treatment. Always seek the advice of your physician or other qualified health provider with any questions you may have regarding a medical condition, including without limitation diabetes. Never disregard professional medical advice or delay in seeking it because of something you have read on TuDiabetes. All views on living with diabetes that are posted on this website are based on personal experiences. (TuDiabetes, 2016, Disclaimer section, para. 1.)

Although this editorial policy does not use the phrase *for me,* the intent of the language is the same. As a grassroots organization, founded by and staffed by people with diabetes, this policy parenthetically adds this phrase to anything anyone posts. As a rhetorical strategy, this hedging also embodies the medical principle of doing no harm and, as such, further aligns the people giving advice in the online community with health care professional identities.

EVALUATING OTHER EXPERTS

Another way people with diabetes establish professional identities is by evaluating medical and scientific information in the form of cure scams and evaluating the expertise of medical professionals. In the evaluative statements diabetics make about site interlopers (i.e., people advertising *cures* on the website), they often mimic the same evaluative stance providers use to discuss patients.

> NIKKI: I think one of the other things that are a big no-no to have on these boards is trying to talk about a cure—and I don't just mean the hope of finding a cure or discussing new studies that could potentially bring about a cure; I mean people that get on there and say, "oh, just follow this raw diet and it'll cure your diabetes," or, "these are the ways for you to lose weight and exercise and this will cure your diabetes," or, "take this supplement 20 times a day and, you know, it'll knock down your blood sugars and cure your diabetes." And, man, there are a lot of people that do that and every once in awhile you get a rash of people that get in and try to, I don't know. I expect that they're not diabetics and they get on there and try to tell people they should do these things or they're trying to push some kind of supplement or thing or whatever. You know, you should never give false hopes to other people.

The members of my other focus group had the following exchange:

> GRACE: It's funny that you say that, because on *Diabetes Daily*, on the Facebook page, there was a guy that came in a couple of days ago claiming that he used to be on like 90 units of insulin a day. He's had diabetes 20 years and he claimed that he's no longer on insulin. So I'm being coy right now and kind of been corresponding back and forth to him, saying, "I'm really excited about getting off of insulin," and I'm waiting to see what he says, but he writes like he's got verbal diarrhea of the fingertips. He really talks out a lot. So it's interesting.
> CONNIE: It's all in his book for only $39.95!
> GRACE: I know, I know. He almost sounds like he could be a good K-tel, you know, "slice it, dice it, and you'll get rid of your diabetes!"
> DAVID: "For two easy payments of $19.95!"

Nikki's positions herself as an expert because she knows this is a fake cure. She does not seem to base this insight on her own experience (Nikki is a type 2), but on her understanding of the physiological processes of the disease and what can or cannot work to treat the disease, specialized knowledge that a medical specialist would possess. She also uses cure discourse that is associated with type 1 diabetes and is evident in public discourse such as on the

Juvenile Diabetes Research Foundation's website, as in the names of events including the Ride to Cure Diabetes and Kids Walk to Cure Diabetes, events that occur across the country annually. Nikki, however, co-opts this discourse to express her skepticism about the notion of there being a cure for the disease, a skepticism readily assumed by many in the diabetic community. In fact, within the community, people often talk about a so-called conspiracy theory that a cure will never happen because pharmaceutical companies make too much money off of people with diabetes. The language surrounding type 2 generally uses the term *reversing* your diabetes rather than curing it. The playful exchange between Connie, Grace, and David uses reported speech to question the credibility of these *scammers,* much in the way medical providers use reported speech when questioning the credibility of patients. In other words, people with diabetes mimic not only a rhetorical strategy but also an authoritative position in relation to someone else. Nikki, Connie, Grace, and David police the activity of these people online, a behavior that mimics the behavior of medical professionals interested in having patients with diabetes comply with conventional medical treatment.

A similar evaluation of real medical providers (rather than *scammers*) appears in the reported speech of people with diabetes. In these reports, the person is clearly positioned as a professional rather than simply parroting the advice given to them by an expert. This pattern occurred in the responses by newly diagnosed participants as well as people who had been diabetic for a number of years. Through reported speech, Tom and Paige directly question the expertise of medical providers as well as emphasizing their own expertise.

> TOM: I would also say find a doctor who is going to hold you to a pretty high standard, who is not going to let you slack. Not someone who is going to say, "Oh, your A1C, that's not too bad. That's fine. You have to live." Find health care professionals that are going to motivate you to manage the disease as best you can. Don't find people who are going to be okay with fair levels of control because that was acceptable maybe twenty years ago and that's when they were trained.

When Paige spoke of questioning the authority of medical providers in chapter 4, she used reported speech:

> I mean, I have met on the internet a large number of people who are having much lower carb diets than the so-called recommendations for diabetics, and the medical profession as a whole doesn't seem to be acknowledging the value of that, but it works for a ton of people. So, if you know something

like that you go in better armed than if you say, "I'm just going to do exactly what you say, doctor."

Tom uses nonspecialized language in the reported speech from a physician. Rather than using specific A1C numbers in this speech, Tom uses the words "not too bad" and "that's fine." The person in conversation with Tom immediately draws a mental image of a doctor who is lazy and/or not up to date in the literature of the disease. The provider, therefore, is discredited as an expert. Paige's reported speech approaches the subject a bit differently. Using her own reported speech to a doctor, she provides an option for patients to go into a doctor's appointment with enough knowledge to have a discussion about care rather than a lecture in which the patient simply, almost childishly, says "I'm just going to do exactly what you say, doctor."

In some ways, these expressions of professional identities could be attributed to the process of protoprofessionalization as discussed in the field of mental health by de Swaan (1981), who has characterized such protoprofessionalization as a process that

> transforms laymen into rudimentary professionals, with an elementary awareness of what a profession deals with, what its basic concepts and occupational stances are, so that these laymen may then employ the same notions to orient themselves in everyday life, to categorize everyday troubles as problems that are suitable for treatment by this or that profession. (p. 359)

Hak and de Boer (1996) describe such protoprofessionalization as a process that occurs as psychotherapists paraphrase patients' speech in their sessions. The reported speech used by people with diabetes, however, has richer consequences than that of such protoprofessionalization because both identification and mimesis are about more than copying or mimicking. Burke (1950) suggests that in the process of identification we continually seek association with certain individuals (and not others), partly to attain some position in the hierarchy of social relations. Rhetorical scholars also caution that the intent of mimesis is not to copy but to surpass. In fact, Corbett (1971) regrets the fact that rhetoricians used the verb imitate, denoting "to produce an image of," for this activity, offering the Latin verb aemu-lari, which means "to try to rival or equal or surpass" as a better choice (p. 244). Terrill (2011) puts it this way: "Imitatio is not a single-minded process in which the rhetor simply absorbs and then regurgitates another's ideas, but a double-minded inventive process through which the student rhetor analyzes both the model text and the target situation in order to craft discourse fitted to her purposes, abilities, and audience" (p. 302). In other words, because patients articulate lived experience and professional discourse, they surpass medical professionals as experts, which would argue for the prefix *para,* which means "side by side," to be attached to *professional* rather than *proto,* which indicates a beginner.

MIMICKING SCIENTIFIC EXPERT PRACTICES

Along with these instances of evaluating information from doctors to patients, people with diabetes evaluate scientific information in a way that repeats some of the practices of scientists: participating in the peer review process and engaging in experiments. Many of the diabetics interviewed for this study talked about reading information on medical websites and in medical journals. Sam, for example, said,

> I read what's for free. I hooked up with Johns Hopkins and Mayo, and I get emailed every day from those people. Some of it is junk, and some of it I read as much as they'll give me for free. They're all selling a $14.95 paper that they spend most of their time telling you how much you're going to get out of it, rather than the facts of the study.

Liz also reads the medical journals:

> A lot of people come to me for advice and mentorship, and I try to be there for folks when they have questions. I don't see myself as diabetes expert in any way. I'm not good at memorizing studies or reading all kinds. I mean, I may read the journals, I do read them. I have them in the back of my mind here and there, but I'm not great at quoting studies to people on different things off the top of my head all the time. But I'm good for helping people know most of what I know about whatever their question is.

Other people with diabetes also call upon evidence they have read in the peer-reviewed scholarship when talking about a recurring debate about names in the online diabetes community. In her 2010 article in the *Chicago Tribune,* Julie Deardorff called this activity the "diabetes' civil war." Some of my interviewees referred to it as the "diabetes smackdown," briefly discussed in chapter 1. In the controversy that flared up over a recent call to change the names of type 1 and type 2 in the petition uploaded to Change.org, people commenting on the site often got into tussles over evidence presented in the peer-reviewed literature as a way to highlight their research gravitas:

Do you follow the professional journals and read about the research? I don't think Type 1 is put on the back burner at all. It may be true that the popular media focus more on Type 2 because a lot of people are at very high risk for it, but back in the universities and research institutes, there are many researchers working on autoimmunity in general, and Type 1 diabetes in particular.

But just as interestingly, because the petition asks decision makers at the ADA (American Diabetes Association), NIH (National Institutes of Health) and IDF (International Diabetes Federation) to revise the names of both type 1 and type 2 diabetes to more accurately reflect the nature of each disease, the mothers who wrote the petition are participating in the scientific practice of defining the disease. They state that the medical community should determine appropriate names, as those professionals are the most qualified; but just as an example, they offer that the unique nature of type 1 would be reflected in a name such as Autoimmune Beta Cell Apoptosis (BCA) Diabetes and the unique nature of type 2 in a name such as Insulin Resistance Diabetes (IRD).

The very fact that people with diabetes and parents of children with diabetes participate in a scientific process of naming suggests that they inhabit a scientific ethos. We can see the penchant to classify in medicine in terms of the diagnostic classifications in the *Diagnostic and Statistical Manual of Mental Disorders* (DSM), the International Statistical Classification of Diseases and Related Health Problems codes (ICD-10 codes) used in medical billing, and, of course, the ADA's *Standards of Medical Care* for the diagnosis and treatment of diabetes. McCarthy (1991) and those following her work with the various updates to the DSM classifications system perhaps most famously reported on this process of classification in the area of mental health.[7]

In the online discussions about the need for change (or the need for no change), people with diabetes participate in similar classification activities. For instance, diabetes blogger Lee Ann Thill had this to say:

The problem with not really understanding the diseases [type 1 and type 2] is that a name you assign today might be proven to be a misnomer with future research findings. I've heard some people suggest that type 1 be called auto-immune diabetes, or something to that effect, and I'd made the suggestion myself back when I thought the name change was a good idea. However, did you know there's research evidence that there is an auto-immune reac-

7. See McCarthy and Gerring (1994); Berkenkotter (2001); and Berkenkotter and Ravotas (1997).

tion involved in the development of type 2 diabetes? My point is that coming up with descriptive names, as opposed to the current generic, symbolic names is highly problematic when you have diseases that need to be further researched, which have some differences, but also have a lot of similarities.

The controversy continues in the comment to Thill's post, and at one point one of the women who created the petition weighs in to clarify. Another commenter, referring to the two suggestions the women offer for new names, says:

Your two immediate suggestions don't really help clarify anything. As Lee Ann mentioned in her post, type 2 diabetes has recently been shown to have autoimmune elements. And Beta Cell death occurs in both type 1 and type 2 diabetes, to varying degrees.

At this point, the conversation shifts to one between the petition creator and the blogger, Thill, arguing for who has done their scientific research. Thill retorts:

I read the entire petition before writing my own piece about it. I maintain that another name change will not really change anything. . . . What if it's discovered that there aren't two distinct types? Maybe there are more than just two types, or maybe there are two types, but one or both have subtypes? As stated in my post, the continued lack of scientific understanding about the nature of both diseases as understood in 2013 means that any possible name change could ultimately be yet more misnomers. Research has shown evidence that there is an autoimmune process at work in type 2, so calling type 1 auto-immune something or other could be as confusing as calling it IDDM—neither names truly differentiate t1 from t2. What about people with type 1 who develop insulin resistance as they age? You state in your petition that type 1 is characterized by rapid beta cell destruction, what about people who develop type 1 as adults, whose beta cell destruction is much slower, and differential diagnosis is more complicated? I've known adults who present as LADA, but the results of their antibody tests are unclear.

Jamie Perez, one of the petition writers, replies:

Our intent is to clear the confusion surrounding both types of D that don't have a name. Our hope for T2s is that they take a name revision such as Insulin Resistance D (IRD) and use it as a platform to explain how the resistance is what has resulted in D, but there are so many factors that can lead to insulin resistance. Our hope is that they publicize the fact that the resistance can be attributable to lifestyle. BUT it isn't always- that it can be attributed to things such as genetics, bio-chemical reactions, POCS [polycystic ovary syndrome], etc. I also want to mention that we, too, came across the immune responses involvement in T2. We originally thought that Autoimmune Diabetes would be a good example for T1, but we found a lot of recent research pointing to an immune response involved in T2- not an immune response on the part of the pancreas or as a direct cause, but as part of the process. As you mentioned, they are finding that excess fat around cells can lead to an immune response against those cells that leads to the insulin resistance. So insulin resistance is still the direct cause of T2- thus our name example for T2. But autoimmune wasn't good enough alone to distinguish T1 so we clarified that the action resulted in beta cell apoptosis (which means cell death). We chose the exact example we used for T1 because the very term Autoimmune Beta Cell Apoptosis is actually used in many recent medical papers, studies and presentations to refer to T1. . . .

What is most interesting in this exchange is how the language takes on aspects of directives much like the provider interviewees used in their reported speech rather than the hedging language often used when scientists talk peer to peer (Hyland, 1996; MacDonald, 2005) or the hedging language people with diabetes use with other diabetics. The language does not include verbs like *suggest*, rather *research has shown* and *we thought* and *found*. The use of such words contains a level of certainty scientists do not use when addressing peers, but do use when writing for lay audiences (Fahnestock, 1986), which would seem to indicate that the individuals in this discussion are not authorities and that scientific ethos by mimesis in this case is unsuccessful, producing an inferior copy of the original. This distinction does, however, echo the established hierarchy discussed in chapter 1 between science, applied medicine (i.e., the practice of medicine rather than medical research), and patients and publics. Unlike the people with diabetes and the providers in my focus groups and interviews who discussed the relationship between fellow diabetics as a mentoring one, the people in the conversations around changing the names of type 1 and type 2 diabetes are engaged in knowledge production. MacDonald (2005) discusses language used to indicate knowledge production in her article about the varying language in journalistic accounts and scientific accounts of hormone replacement news. She suggests that journalism genres sensationalize scientific communication because of the language conventions used by the genre. These conventions include the class of sentence subject (a person versus data or research) and the use of concrete verbs. Journalism, for example, might use "Jenny Smith took hormones" whereas scientific writing would use "Data indicated that . . ." (MacDonald, 2005, p. 280). MacDonald attributes these differences to a distinction between writing that focuses on "the phenomena themselves" and writing that focuses on "its own epistemic methods" (2005, p. 279). Writing that focuses on "the phenomena themselves" (MacDonald, 2005, p. 279) foregrounds individuals and human actors. Writing that focuses on "its own epistemic methods" foregrounds data and knowledge. On the other hand, the language also mimics the providers' directive reported speech and the directive language used on organization websites and in the ADA *Standards of Medical Care* document. Together, this form of mimesis, therefore, does indicate a similar positioning between medical providers and people with diabetes.

Another way people with diabetes position themselves as medical authorities online is through mimicking the structure of a question format one might encounter with filling out a medical history form or in the verbal exchange that takes place in a traditional doctor visit: "How many times a day do you test? Are you on MDI? I test a lot, so if I see a bad number, I can catch it before it gets worse." Others discredit doctors:

1. Find a new doctor, quickly. You need the blood work done. Your doctor should have done something for this. I have found with me it takes 3 weeks minimum for meds to kick in and bring my BG levels down and you are way past that.
2. Have you been to any education classes or seen a nutritionist? Will your insurance provide these for you? I think you need to be better educated about what this disease can do to you if it is not controlled and you are in the position right now to take control. If you do not you will be sorry. Yes, more doom and gloom but . . . I hope you read Lois' story, I have two more for you if you want. They're not pretty.

Finally, people with diabetes mimic scientific ethos through using experimentation as a method of discovery in their participation in and discussion of clinical trials.

TOM: I still don't know if I was a placebo or if I received the active drug. I didn't really notice any big improvement. We always had infusions on Tuesdays. There's three sequential infusions of this stem cell agent, one month apart. For that week, maybe until the next Tuesday, I noticed I was going lower a lot, so I had to back down my [basal] insulin level, so maybe it had some short-term or transient benefit, but always I would creep back up to pretreatment levels. I don't think it had any long-term impacts.

Rick, another focus group participant, echoed this practice:

You know, a place that I've learned that's kind of nontraditional is in diabetic trials. For most of my life I have tried to do diabetic trials whenever possible, and it's amazing . . . the usual stuff you hear during the trials that later becomes gospel in the diabetic community, and I find that to be a place that I go to find information.

Discussing the discourse of stem cell technology, Lynch (2011) argues that political discourse borrows language from science and scientific authorities to make arguments. He says that "scientistic idioms," the rhetorical strategies and arguments associated with science that become part of public debate, do more than just mimic science to create "an illusion of understanding" (Lynch, 2011, p. 4). Instead, they create real definitions from which people can make sense of the world and argue for specific actions. As the examples in this chapter show, people with diabetes use scientific language when communicating in liminal spaces (i.e., group spaces of health), and thus create a similarly real definition of themselves as professionals. In doing so, people with diabetes are doing what medical professionals and scholars of medical and health rhetoric have not been able to do: They have positioned themselves *within* the work places of health and medicine. Of course, not all health care spaces are liminal, and the traditional doctor office visit is not likely to be completely replaced by group appointments. Therefore, this positioning within liminal spaces can have important implications for other spaces in health that require people to engage in dialogues about their care. Increasingly, the institution of medicine has been focusing on creating such a dialogue in the spaces in which providers practice. To fully engage in such a partnership requires patients to do more than come in to their doctor appointments with what one physician described to me as their Dr. Oz list, a list of concerns and questions a patient creates and brings to a medical appointment. They also need to do more than just bring lived experience into the exam room. They need to develop a professional voice in these encounters. Making use of mimesis is one way to do that. Patients can bring in the voice of other expert patients, for example. In a time when we are skeptical about traditional expertise and people will often prefer information from a peer over that of an established authority (Weinberger, 2012), this rhetorical strategy might shift the dynamic from one-sided persuasion to a dialog or negotiated decision. As such, expert patients can perform agency in spaces that have not been generative for this kind of work in the past.

Re-Articulating Agency and Looking to Patient-Centered Changes

AS WITH most problems that are difficult to solve because of incomplete or contradictory knowledge, varied opinions, and interconnections with other problems, locating agency in diabetes requires a complex approach such as the re-mapping project undertaken here. The re-articulations presented offer a definition of patient agency that have implications for how agency is theorized in the rhetoric of health and medicine. Furthermore, these re-articulations enrich the medical community's description of patient agency in both liminal and nonliminal spaces and complicate agency in ways that can be useful to technical and medical communicators, medical providers, and, ultimately, people with diabetes.

IMPLICATIONS FOR THE RHETORIC OF HEALTH AND MEDICINE

When compliance's hold on interpretations of agency in diabetes discourse is loosened and other articulations become possible, agency can be redefined as a relational and performative act. This agency, like that described by Hauser and Kjeldsen (2010) in relation to vernacular discourse, "involves each member of society as a *point of articulation* who invents his or her agential capacity moment-by-moment through everyday exchanges" (p. 95; emphasis in original). In collaborative spaces, such as those under discussion here, disparate discourses are juxtaposed and these articulations and re-articulations are negotiated through a capacity to form a number of constellations that have consequences for how agency is theorized.

In conversations about agency in institutions with the potential for extreme power differentials, scholars have often come back to the agency/structure problem and representations of agency as an individual force within a framework of domination. In many ways, this theory of agency aligns with ideas about autonomy that resonate with traditional medical definitions of patient agency. Such a view has been popular in social movement rhetoric such as that of disabilities studies and some feminist movements. Proponents of the social model of disability have argued that people with disabilities are an oppressed group because society's actions exclude and isolate them from fully participating in society (Shakespeare, 2006). Although feminism includes numerous ideologies, a fundamental claim of feminism is that women are oppressed and "feminism is the struggle to end sexist oppression" (hooks, 2000). Much of the political strength of such cohesive social movements is in their acts of resistance, but the contemporary patient as a socially bound or motivated single group united in a single action is as fictional as the public Grabill and Simmons discuss (1998). Therefore, seeing patients as an organized force of social resistance to oppressive forces is counterproductive and reinforces the problematic view of people with diabetes as a singular patient set.

In discourses of health care it may be more productive to view the relationship between power and resistance as a complex network with "multiple points of potential difference or divergence bringing possibilities for disruption to the discursive flow" (Armstrong & Murphy, 2012, p. 322). Most often such disruption is seen as the end project of agency: Agential acts create positive change.[1] As the findings here show, change, in the form of the ability to re-articulate multiple materials, discourses, identities, and subjectivities, is a resource for rather than a result of agency. Agency emerges as a rhetorical response in this network of situated practices as diabetics enact identities as experts and novices, draw upon various types of knowledge, and employ this knowledge and subjectivity through a continual process of discursive maneuvers. This characterization of the relationship between agency and change comes through in chapter 2 in the counter narratives people with diabetes generate and chapter 3 in the discussion of diabetics' relationships with knowledge and the ongoing choices they make in terms of which type of knowledge

---

1. See, for example, Enck-Wanzer (2006) and Sowards (2010).

to use or share. The characterization continues in chapter 4's discussion of multiple subjectivities and the ways that people with diabetes shift between expert and novice subjectivities in their interactions with other diabetics and is evident as mimesis as discussed in chapter 5.

In relation to the powerful discourse of the biomedical industrial complex, complicating the structure-agency dichotomy has implications for agency in other situations in which players are marginalized and power is at issue. Of course, this entire book focuses on moving our understanding of agency forward as it applies to the subject at hand. In studies of agency in other health contexts, however, two questions can act as a heuristic for creating rhetorically grounded understandings of health and disease that will facilitate our understandings of the cultural forms of other chronic diseases.

1. What articulations are currently enacted?
2. What alternate articulations are possible?

For this project, asking these questions has resulted in a shift in understanding agency as a top-down concept (figure 4) to a dynamic and somewhat messy one (figure 5).

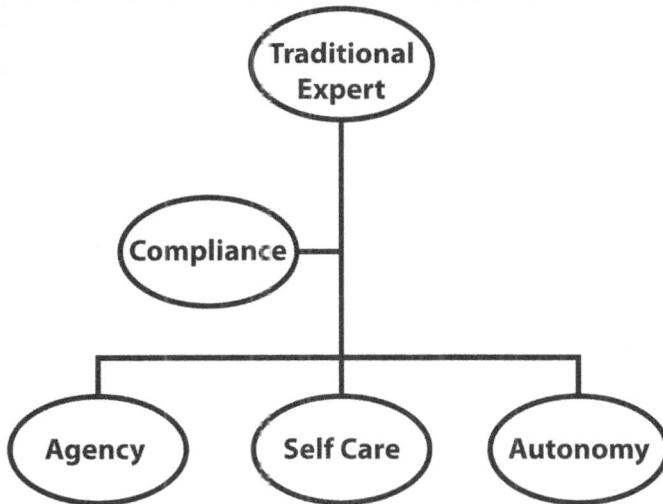

FIGURE 4. A linear model of agency. Image from Daisy Allen Cunningham.

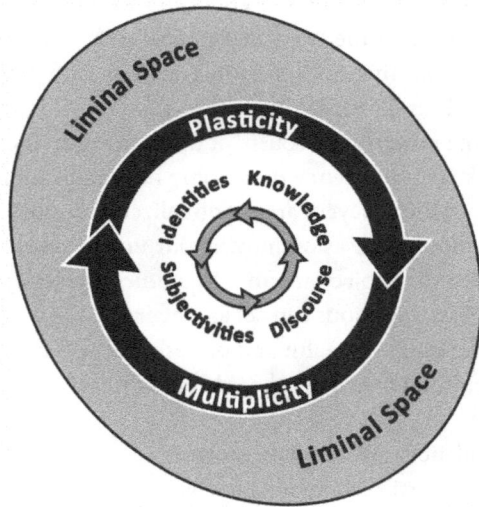

FIGURE 5. An alternative model for agency. Image from Daisy Allen Cunningham.

RE-ARTICULATING THE LANGUAGE AND PRACTICES OF MEDICINE IN DIABETES

Along with adding to our body of knowledge about agency in health and medical contexts, this project has what Segal (2005) would refer to as useful implications or what Miller (1989a) might call practical consequences, which involve how patient-centered care gets delivered in the twenty-first century. In 2001, the Institute of Medicine declared that patient-centered care would become one of its six focal points in improving care (2001a, p. 6); since health care has been trying to evolve away from a disease-centered model and toward a patient-centered model in which patients become active participants in their care (Institute of Medicine, 2001b). Still, there is little to no consensus on the definition of patient-centered care, much less on what it looks like in practice. This study, grounded in rhetorical theory and technical communication practices, moves the discussion about patient-centered care forward by offering concrete suggestions for creating patient-centered practices, pedagogies, and texts.

Patient-Centered Practices

This project has implications for the work that gets done in the trenches of medical practices, including the practice of shared decision making. Lying somewhere between paternalistic medicine and autonomous patient actions, shared decision making has four components in theory: (1) it involves at least two participants, (2) all participants participate in the process of treatment decision making, (3) it includes information sharing, and (4) all parties agree on the treatment decision (Charles, Gafni, & Whelan, 1997). Shared decision making in medicine is largely informed by decision science, which Miller (1989b) describes as a theory of choice with its origin in economic theory. It relies on mathematical logarithms that generate personalized sets of data about a patient, such as their risk factors for stroke (i.e., high blood pressure, age, and gender). Using this information, a physician and a patient examine and compare treatment alternatives (typically prescription medication), one of which will, it is presumed, emerge as a correct, even obvious, choice. For example, in treating a common heart condition known as atrial fibrillation, an irregular and often rapid heartbeat that causes poor blood flow to the body, doctors often talk to patients about anticoagulation treatment such as Warfarin. These conversations take place because a complication of atrial fibrillation is stroke. Taking anticoagulation medication decreases this likelihood, but it comes with its own set of risk factors: Patients on anticoagulation therapy are at risk for bleeding events, particularly gastrointestinal bleeding.

In this decision-making interaction, doctors share scientific evidence while patients share values and preferences. As currently practiced, however, shared decision making aligns with a deficit model of communication, a view similar to the transmission model Slack et al. (1993) discussed or the conduit metaphor offered by Shannon and Weaver (1948), which moves information from a transmitter to a receiver. The use of this language enforces the binary of expert and lay person, relegating the lay person's expertise to doxa, which is often put in contrast to episteme. Whereas episteme concerns things that can be objectively and scientifically proved, doxa concerns opinions and beliefs. This misses the fact that patients do not accept information as is, as Paige and other people with diabetes so clearly illustrate throughout this book. At the same time, it privileges *some* forms of logic and rational decisions, making the assumption that all patients will be swayed by evidence that comes from medical authorities. As the data in this study show, however, sharing information and truly participating in a decision-making process are not necessarily one in the same. The model of agency presented here could help to change this dynamic and encourage more medical professionals to practice shared decision making as Montori, Gafni, and Charles (2006) define it. They argue for a model in which the patient gathers and shares technical information and the clinician, who "come[s] from different cultural or socio-economical worlds or hold different world views (resulting from clinicians' training and experience)" brings his or her values and preferences to the interaction (Montori et al., 2006, p. 32). In other words, they argue for somewhat reversing the roles of patients and clinicians in these encounters by having both parties exchange both information and preferences.

Based on the data presented in this book, like Montori et al. (2006), I want to suggest that the partnership between the so-called clinical team and the health care team needs to include other people with diabetes as group appointments and online patient communities do. One way this can happen in traditional appointments with just the doctor and patient is through the patient bringing in the voice of other expert patients through reported speech, as in the reported speech moments discussed in the preceding chapter. For example, in meetings I participate in with a group of physicians, people present their research projects in order get feedback. In these presentations, they regularly draw on a hypothesized patient as a form of reported speech to explain their ideas in more concrete detail by way of example. This is a naturally occurring pattern in these meetings. If physicians drew on similar hypothetical patients in their shared decision-making appointments with their own patients, they could draw on identification through mimesis as a resource for making co-produced treatment decisions.

Educating patients how to use reported speech could be fruitful as well. Advocacy organizations such as the American Diabetes Association could explain how to talk to a physician in this manner in the educational materials they provide for people on their website rather than telling them to write down and bring a list of questions to their doctor. Whereas writing these lists of questions and exercises like writing goals on the handout with the ladder image I discussed in chapters 2 and 4 are designed to instill agency, the result is not agential. By invoking reported speech as a rhetorical strategy, however, patients can bring not only their own voices and lived experiences to these encounters but the voices and logics from a variety of experts. It also shifts subjectivities for both the patient and physician. Rather than the patient being a student with questions and the doctor a teacher with knowledge, both patient and physician engage in a dialog, which can result the reaching a truly shared decision.

Patient-Centered Pedagogies

Patient-centered pedagogies are important for people living with chronic illness like diabetes because they do need to be trained to do the work of their disease management outside of clinical appointments. Diabetes education sessions (both individual and group) tend to default to more traditional models of teaching, such as step instructions or lectures. Of course, it is easy to understand why that path is taken. Medical professionals training for jobs have curricula packed with courses on specialized information they will need to bring to their encounters with patients. These curricula leave little room for conversations about patient-centered pedagogies such as the layered, community-based, or networked models offered here that can be alternatives for medical professionals.

If we think about patient education in terms of the cognitive domain of Bloom's taxonomy (Bloom, Engelhart, Furst, Hill, & Krathwohl, 1956), we can say that medical professionals focus on the three lower regions (knowledge, comprehension, and application) when educating people about diabetes. Bloom's original taxonomy, created in 1956, was designed to promote higher forms of thinking in education rather than just remembering facts. It is typically used for designing educational, training, and learning processes. The committee that created the taxonomy identified three domains of learning: cognitive, affective, and psychomotor. The cognitive domain involves knowledge and includes six major categories: knowledge, comprehension, application, analysis, synthesis, and evaluation. A person is seen as moving up through the lesser domains of remembering facts to evaluating knowledge, then finally creating knowledge. People with diabetes need to learn (and remember) new information and they need to understand it well enough to apply it (i.e., they need to be able to take actions to help control their blood sugar levels).

As the data in this study have repeatedly shown, however, people with diabetes also enact the three higher levels (analyzing, evaluating, and creating). Therefore, less step-focused or linear models of the learning process can be more useful in diabetes educational settings. More satisfying models can be found in technical communication pedagogy. Such models of technical communication pedagogy make agency a major concern. Cook's (2002) framework of layered literacies, for example, includes basic, rhetorical, social, technological, ethical, and critical literacies. Cook argues that these literacies are necessary for the multiple ways technical communicators need to solve complex problems through language. Cook's inclusion of basic literacy is reminiscent of linear approaches to learning, but the other five literacies are interwoven in terms of learning to problem solve through language. The people with diabetes in this study certainly draw on all these literacies. As they shift expert subjectivities they do so according to the audiences they interact with, showing rhetorical skills of understanding the audience's role in shaping their expertise. Through metis they draw on technological literacies to hack technology and make it work better. They make ethical choices in their everyday decisions that impact their health. Finally, they are able "to recognize and consider ideological stances and power structures" (Cook, 2002, p. 16) and yet still be willing to help others in need, as they do in online and face-to-face group settings.

A pedagogy informed by such rhetorical, social, and critical literacies involves collaborative work. Cook (2002) reminds us that research in workplace practices has demonstrated the crucial role social skills play in technical communicators' success in terms of collaboration and as a part of the writing process in most workplaces. As such, another solution/model we might draw on for educational work in diabetes group settings is that of a community of practice, a community in which members are practitioners who "develop a shared repertoire of resources: experiences, stories, tools, ways of addressing recurring problems—in short a shared practice." (Wenger, 2006, "Practice" section, para. 1).[2] The community itself has an identity defined by a shared interest, and members pursue this interest through joint activities and discussions.

Networked pedagogies also have been identified as a successful strategy for workplace topographies in which the flow of information is increasingly fluid, as opposed to the one-way flow of information the medical neighborhood represents. Learning in these environments occurs horizontally, peripherally, nomadically, and independently (Bay, 2010). Horizontal learning happens across boundaries rather than through vertical hierarchies. In this type of networked learning, individuals are constantly developing multiple skills sets and are shifting between multiple roles, much like the people with diabetes in this project. In networked learning environments, a student would learn from other students (as people with diabetes learn from each other) as well as other resources including, but not limited to, the teacher. Peripheral learning in these spaces occurs on the edges of classroom practice. It might be in the form of in-person or virtual study groups, for example. In student settings, nomadic learning experiences include internships and study abroad experiences. Finally, independent student learning situations are distant in another way, requiring students to work independently and often without direct contact with supervisors and established workplace environments. This kind of activity already emerges organically in online and face-to-face group settings.

Patient-Centered Texts

Although much has changed since Mary Specker Stone (1997) searched for patient agency in the written materials created for patients in the area of

---

2. Arduser (2013a).

managed care, Stone (1997), Bennett (2009 and 2013), and Martins (2005 and 2009) find that what is designed to be patient-centered communication still falls short. One reason for this is that the production of educational materials for people with diabetes is an undertaking that often does not include people with diabetes in the development process.[3] When I interviewed the director of the NDEP several years ago, for example, she explained the process of developing the educational resources the organization produced. The materials went through a revision process that included getting feedback from people in high-risk groups for type 2 diabetes (African Americans, Native Americans, Asian Americans, and Pacific Islanders). However, no material was examined by people with the disease. Curious to see what feedback such an audience might offer, I later worked with students in a graduate usability class at Texas Tech University where the students developed and ran a usability test that included people with diabetes. The testing group totaled six users, including two users who had diabetes, two users who had family members with diabetes, and two users who had not been diagnosed with diabetes nor had family members with diabetes. In the test, the students divided the original "4 Steps to Control Your Diabetes for Life" pamphlet into many independent pieces. The images, headings, and text that were combined in a specific section of the pamphlet were all separated so that each independent piece could be tested for its intuitiveness and understandability out of its original context. Their overall objective was to focus on the message that each image, heading, and block of text conveyed to the user. Each user was also asked to create a new pamphlet, based on the original images, headings, and text, in a way that made the information more understandable to them in order to assess how well the original pamphlet was organized. Their findings suggested that the order of the original pamphlet was not the most useful for its audience (Cole, Hall, Garrison, Ranario, & Tharanathan, n.d.).

The materials I examined throughout this book also highlight that the "entrenched language and text conventions of medical professional discourse function to restrain the emergence of patient agency" (Stone, 1997, p. 203). Technical communication's attention to what Robert Johnson (1997) called *audience involved,* however, can give the diabetes medical community a concept to draw into their own practices of developing educational materials. This concept of *audience involved* goes one step further than networked learning in that students are not just learning from but also creating knowledge that can, in turn, help determine the content of the discourse. Johnson (1997) says, "The involved audience brings the audience literally into the open, making the

---

3. This exclusion is reminiscent of the omission of patients in the medical neighborhood as discussed in chapter 2.

intended audience a visible, physical, collaborative presence" (p. 363). Moving from audiences to end users, Johnson says that technical communicators cannot just be user advocates but must involve actual users in the production process. Johnson's concept of *audience involved* particularly resonates in rethinking collaboration in a time of the maker movement; a do-it-yourself, or DIY, ethos; and a prosumer culture. In terms of this research, we can see this ethos in action in the practices of Patient-Centered Outcomes Research Institute (PCORI), a nonprofit, nongovernmental organization established in accordance with the Patient Protection and Affordable Care Act of 2010, which similarly included patients *upstream* in the process of research. The group encourages patient input through a variety of mechanisms, including submitting research questions they would like PCORI to consider for funding as well as providing formal public comment on draft reports, policies, and initiatives; reviewing research applications; and participating on advisory panels.

This new model of patient agency offered in this book has several entry points for making patient-centered changes to the texts. One such entry point involves changes in the communication practices in group appointments. While these are designed to be spaces that value everyone's knowledge, they also maintain ties to a compliance-based framework that works through an expert dispensing knowledge to a novice and, as such, operate with a diminished view of agency. Agency practiced through different rhetorical strategies in these spaces could be more patient centered. For example, in one of my graduate classes, students developed educational materials to help people with type 1 diabetes. The students created an e-book for people with type 1 transitioning from their parents' home to workplaces and college.[4]

The e-book moves from internal emotions to physical needs to conversations. It is not designed to teach subject matter knowledge or a skill; it was written to help people gain rhetorical and social literacies that will help them have dialogues with people about the disease, dialogues that do not rely solely on numbers but on their own work as a symbolic analyst. Understanding what agency looks like and how it is enacted can be particularly useful in large transitions like that between adolescence and adulthood, but it is also useful for the smaller, ceaseless changes with this disease, whether it is the change from gestational diabetes to type 2 diabetes or moving from taking insulin shots to using an insulin pump. Using this book in group appointment settings, people could role-play the various conversations the book describes. One person

---

4. Because type 1 often develops in childhood, parents play a large role in self-management and communicating to people about their child's disease. As children enter adulthood, transitioning these responsibilities can be difficult for both the person with diabetes and the parent.

could be the new worker with diabetes, for instance, and the other person the impatient, uninformed boss.

Shared decision-making texts offer another entry point.[5] These tools are used across a range of disciplines and decision points—from statin choice to hip replacement surgery to taking antibiotics for bronchitis (Sorrell, 2014).[6] They might be in the form of brochures, videos, websites, or cards. The Mayo Clinic Shared Decision Making National Resource Center website, for example, offers tools to help people make single-episode decisions about medication. These texts, focus on a single decision that needs to be made at a single point in time, such as deciding which type of blood pressure medicine to take when hypertension is first diagnosed, and a single condition and, as such, do not take into consideration the permanent liminality of chronic illness decision making. Treatment decisions that involve patients with chronic conditions need to be made and revisited on an ongoing basis. People with chronic illnesses grapple with illness over an extended period of time; the condition is subject to change and may include multiple conditions or diseases that need to be taken into account rather than just the one disease and one treatment option at hand. In these chronic settings there needs to be an ongoing partnership between the clinician and the patient because there are multiple windows of opportunity, and choices can be revisited and even reversed over long periods of time.

Given that diabetes is a permanent liminal state in and of itself, other, more interactive tools may also be useful in negotiating the material of agency. Like the users in the interactive data displays that Rawlins and Wilson (2014) discuss, people with diabetes are interpretive, creative agents. They participate in the creation of the decision, the knowledge, and the identities constructed in their interactions with other people with diabetes and health care professionals. As such, an interactive shared decision-making tool might look something like the experience maps used in user experience work in technical communication.

These maps present a longitudinal version of what researchers in technical communication call personas.[7] Personas are often used in developing products as a form of audience analysis. A development team will create a set of perso-

<hr>

5. For examples of a variety of shared decision-making tools, see the Mayo Clinic Shared Decision Making National Resource Center website at http://shareddecisions.mayoclinic.org.

6. Statins are a group of drugs that act to reduce levels of triglycerides and cholesterol in the blood.

7. At the 2013 Society for Technical Communication Summit conference, Donn DeBoard presented one such artifact, describing journey maps as tools that visually show a person's entire experience interacting with a company's product. Given my argument against the journey metaphor in chapter 1, I prefer the term *experience map.*

nas that capture demographic and psychographic data of their representative audience. Personas are basically snapshots—a still image in time. As such, they only capture a moment—the diagnosis, the decision to take a particular medication, or the decision to move from insulin injections to an insulin pump. Experience maps move beyond these singular moments as key events and emphasize multiple changes and multiple decisions. Such an outline could be used for a shared decision-making tool. So, for example, typically when a child is diagnosed with type 1 diabetes, the medical team will start that person with insulin shots. After six months or so, a period long enough for the family to adjust to the myriad of changes they are experiencing, the child is likely to go on an insulin pump. A woman with type 1 or 2 might decide it's time to start a family. All of these moments of change require new knowledge and actions. Experience maps could create this biographical outline and be used to inform the design of shared decision-making tools.

In a previous version of the Cornerstones4Care website, Novo Nordisk created navigation that was similar to the idea that drives user experience maps.[8] When a person came to their website, they used photos of people as the next navigational move to get to information specific to them. For example, the speech bullet for one figure said "My diabetes care team just told me I need another medication." Other figures say the following:

- I'm just looking for information right now.
- I'm not happy with my diabetes care program.
- I'm doing okay managing my diabetes, but I want to do better.
- I have or care for someone with type 1 diabetes.
- My doctor just told me that I have diabetes.

This website is particularly successful at negotiating some of the agential agency discussed throughout this book. As with all of the other texts designed for people with diabetes, two of the figures on this website rely on classification (of type 1 diabetes, in this case) and on the moment of diagnosis as a point of intervention. The other four figures, however, address topics that are not often presented. As my interviewees and focus group participants with diabetes described in chapter 4, people often feel like nonexperts at different times than just the point of diagnosis. These entry points for information on the website capture this nuance of living with the disease.

---

8. The current website is different, but this version can be viewed at https://web.archive .org/web/20120629092216/http://www.cornerstones4care.com/.

If we think of the experience map as something that tracks the articulations people with diabetes make with their bodies, medical providers, and other diabetics, such a map might prove useful based on its focus on a diachronic outline of a user's experience (Howard, 2014). This shift could be an alternative for the spatial journey metaphor in chronic illness in developing communication tools that can work more effectively over time.

Re-mapping metaphors in patient materials used in these settings could also play a role in revising texts to be more patient-centered. Nearly forty years ago, Susan Sontag (1978) began the conversation about the way metaphors attach themselves to certain diseases and influence attitudes toward those who experience the disease. Some of the metaphors used for chronic illness have not changed since Sontag's essays were published. However, Hanne and Hawken's (2007) study of metaphors used in news articles about avian flu, cancer, diabetes, heart disease, and HIV/AIDS in *The New York Times* concluded that while the diseases Sontag wrote of (cancer and HIV/AIDS) still appear, they attract "far fewer, and less alarmist, metaphors" (p. 94) than those used with avian flu and diabetes. Hanne and Hawken surmise that this phenomenon is caused in part by the fact that cancer and HIV/AIDS are better understood and more effectively treated. The metaphors they found associated with diabetes include military phrases such as "one day in the trenches" (a reference to a visit to a diabetes ward); "genetics may load the cannon, but human behavior pulls the trigger"; "bombarded with all the societal influences"; and "a forced death march" (Hanne & Hawken, 2007, p. 96). They also found metaphors for a flood or storm, such as a "huge wave of new cases" and repeated use of the term "surge" for the rising incidence of diabetes (Hanne & Hawken, 2007, p. 96).[9]

Within medical discourse about chronic illness, metaphors have tended to focus on three primary constructions: the body as a machine (Lupton, 2003; Segal, 2005), the warfare/military metaphor (Lupton, 2003; Segal, 1997), and medicine as business (Segal, 1997). Specifically within diabetes care, metaphors often tend to characterize the disease as a journey, as the Conversation Maps show. Although for different reasons, however, neither the road/journey metaphor of the Conversation Maps I discussed nor the ladder image in the pharmacists' materials are particularly appropriate for the mode of patient agency described here. The journey metaphor indicates an end. The assumption regarding diabetes is that the end of the game is equal to control being

---

9. Some of this information was reported in the 2013 book chapter "The Care and Feeding of the D-Beast: Metaphors of the Lived Experience of Diabetes" in *Rhetorical Accessibility: At the Intersection of Technical Communication and Disability Studies.*

attained, and since the game (or story) ends, the diabetic thus "lives happily ever after." As the diabetics I interviewed indicate, however, there is no end to this particular journey.

In ways similar to the journey metaphor, the ladder metaphor picks up on characteristics of orientational metaphors, such as *more is up* (the price goes up each year) and *good is up* (things are looking up) (Lakoff & Johnson, 1980). These associations have moral implications that are attached to compliance-based views of agency. Moving to the top step of the ladder (attaining a blood sugar level goal) is *good* and the person that reaches that step is, therefore, a good patient. Such metaphors articulate to activities of acquisition rather than participation. As such, they reflect an ideology of agency as a possession rather than a negotiated performance.

Other metaphors could better reflect agency in the way people with diabetes enact it. For the handout the pharmacists use, for example, a more appropriate metaphor could be a seesaw, communicating the value of balance people with diabetes discuss as well as the ever-changing landscape of blood sugar levels. What becomes apparent in the conversations from this focus group is a definition of control that is more about balance—a state of equilibrium or the power or means to decide—than control. Both providers and people with diabetes have used the term balance but in different ways. Provider web texts use the word in reference to treatments. The ADA and the U.S. Department of Veteran Affairs websites, for example, talk about balancing diet, activity, and medication. The U.S. Department of Veteran Affairs website offers the following:

> Lisa's doctor asked Lisa to do a blood sugar check. To the doctor's surprise, Lisa turned on the timer of her meter before pricking her finger and putting the blood drop on the test strip. The doctor explained to Lisa and her parents that the way Lisa was testing was probably causing the blood sugar test errors. With time, and more accurate blood sugar results, Lisa and her parents got better at using her results to keep food, insulin, and exercise in balance. At later checkups, her blood sugar records and the A1C test results showed good news about her control. (U.S. Department of Veteran Affairs, 2013, A1C Test)

The ADA website uses the term "balance" to talk about the danger of ketones:

> Small or trace amounts of ketones may mean that ketone buildup is starting. You should test again in a few hours. Moderate or large amounts are a

danger sign. They upset the chemical balance of your blood and can poison the body.[10]

In each of these cases, balance is defined in relation to a diabetic treatment plan (balancing diet, exercise, and medication) or balance is seen as a metabolic process. Three participants with diabetes, however, specifically used the term "balance" to refer to a balance between the activities in their lives in general and the disease-related activities rather than a balance of treatments or processes within their body. Ken, who is a support group facilitator and a diabetic himself, uses the term *balance* as a synonym for *control.*

> KEN: Well, it's [control] a personal thing, but I would say that it's an individual's choice on how much effort they're going to place on maintaining their health and balance against the difficulty that they have in making compromises in their life in order to achieve those goals. So, you know, various people tell you about quantitative measures of blood sugar control, and to me, somebody's achieved good control—I think it has to do with achieving a personal balance between the efforts that you make towards your goals in health against the difficulty you have in your life in making those choices. And not everyone's going to have the same set of priorities and make the same set of choices, but hopefully everyone can make choices that will lead them to have a reasonably long and healthy life without having to sacrifice the quality of that life.

Connie and David also used *balance* to refer to the way they alternate between what they do in relation to diabetic care activities and the other things they do in their lives.

> CONNIE: So it's kind of like a balance. You know, it's that perfect balance to live and to live well. And I'm not going to put myself through no-carb living and never have another piece of bread, you know? Just eat cheese and lettuce. I'm not going to do that. Because I plan on living a long, long time, and all those years of eating nothing but cheese and lettuce, you know? I'm going to kill myself. You know?
>
> DAVID: I mean, for certain types of people, micromanaging too much can be stressful. It's definitely a balance. You know, to tell someone, "Well, just

---

10. Copyright © 2013–2015 American Diabetes Association. From: www.diabetes.org. Reprinted with permission from the American Diabetes Association.

write everything down and you'll be fine." You have to be able to look at that data and pull out useful information from it.

Both of these excerpts talk about balance in terms of extreme forms of disease management, a topic that never came up in the provider texts examined here. Connie specifically defines balance as what you do to balance the quality and quantity of life. She refers to a growing segment of the diabetic population who adhere to diet recommendations that suggest eating little to no carbohydrates as a way to control diabetes.[11] David discusses the same extreme behavior in terms of over-monitoring oneself through the activity of keeping a log of all the food a person eats, the exercise the person does, and the medicines a person takes. This myopic view, David suggests, has to be balanced by an analysis of the information being written down. The notion of balance works against the image of the ladder.

Achieving balance may evoke a sense of stability at odds with the picture of agency in diabetes, but in the context of diabetes, achieving balance is an eternal process. If, for example, a person with diabetes eats a slice of birthday cake at her daughter's birthday party, her blood sugar will rise quickly to levels outside of any target range. To swing her levels back to something more acceptable, she might take extra insulin to cover the extra sugar she just ate. Or she might instead go for a run because exercise will bring blood sugar down as well. A few hours later she might need to make some kind of correction gain if she misjudges and takes a little too much insulin or runs a little too long. Because a balance or seesaw has the potential to always be in motion, this metaphor is more appealing than that of stable devices such as a ladder. On the TuDiabetes forums, people talk about balancing their diet and also about balancing their blood sugars when exercising. One person said, "I aim for balance, of course, and that sweet spot where I'm neither high or low, but I think any diabetic knows that balance isn't always possible." Another said, "I like to think of diabetes as being about 'balance' rather than high/low, up/down, good/evil or any of the other ways people think about it."

The metaphor of a journey as a destination with an end or individual exploration similar to the hero's journey does not resonate with the experience of diabetes. The Conversation Maps used in some group appointments could, for example, be constructed in different ways. As currently designed, the Maps focus on the autonomous individual with diabetes. Along the way, diabetics

---

11. The diet was created by Dr. Bernstein, a physician with type 1 diabetes. He advocates for people with diabetes to use a very low carbohydrate diet in order to attain normal, nondiabetic blood glucose numbers. Although patients have been interested in this diet for years, the medical community has only recently talked about using it as a diet strategy.

interact with their own bodies (learning about hypoglycemia and hypergly-cemia), they also interact with relatives and friends as support resources, and they further interact with treatment regimes of diet, exercise, and medica-tions. What is less stressed is the interactions between players (i.e., diabetics) in the room as they move around the Conversation Map board. The develop-ers of the Conversation Maps have made attempts to make these educational materials more interactive. Whereas once they were designed as traditional board games, if a person visits the Journey for Control website in 2016, he will find that these one-dimensional games have been transformed into three-dimensional game simulations. These simulations, however, still lack interac-tions between multiple game players.

The game could be redesigned in several ways to change this. One could play in teams, for instance, or within a virtual world game, an immersive three-dimensional environment in which people use avatars to represent themselves and to move through space (New Media Consortium and EDU-CAUSE Learning Initiative, 2007). The most popular virtual worlds are mul-tiuser spaces in which many people interact within a virtual space in real time (New Media Consortium and EDUCAUSE Learning Initiative, 2007). Characteristics of both game worlds and virtual worlds include several people using shared space, the sense of immediacy, interaction that occurs in real time, interactivity, persistence (the world never shuts down), and community (Araki & Carliner, 2008). These spaces share many of the characteristics I have been discussing in terms of liminality. They, too, involve presence, a charac-teristic related to immediacy and interactivity. Ruggiero, et al. (2014) found this to be the case in their study with the game Diabetes Island. In a study that involved using the Internet-based game with low-income African Americans with type 2 diabetes, the research team found that the participant feedback about the intervention was consistently positive, recommending further study with other populations.

CONCLUSION

My ultimate aim in this book is to argue that an interdisciplinary effort with a foundation in rhetorical theory can drive changes in the discourses and practices of health and medicine. As I have shown, such an approach can dis-articulate patient agency from compliance and re-articulate it to new rela-tionships that are more empowering for people living with chronic disease. In the collaborative spaces examined, agency is a performance that requires a shifting network of elements: knowledge production, subjectivity, and rhetorical strategies. In liminal spaces that juxtapose disparate voices, these articulations and re-articulations are negotiated through a constellation of maneuvers that can be collectively described as a form of rhetorical plasticity. As this project shows, agency emerges as a rhetorical response in this network of situated practices as patients enact identities as experts and novices, draw upon various types of knowledge, and employ this knowledge and subjectivity through a continual process of discursive maneuvers.

These re-articulations also have implications for the health care system. At the beginning of 2016, *The Diane Rehm Show* on National Public Radio interviewed a panel of doctors, health policy experts, and health researchers about doctor-patient communication. While the panel focused on technology and communication, Cindy Brach, a health researcher at the Agency for Healthcare Research and Quality (AHRQ), had this to say about communication in general: "the healthcare system has basically done a pretty—has a pretty poor track record of communicating in writing" (Lakshmanan, 2016, 11:26:53). The majority of such communication efforts have focused on patients' literacy and doctor's bedside manner. As people live longer and live chronic (the number of Americans with diagnosed diabetes alone is projected to increase 165 percent from the year 2000 to 2050 [Boyle, et al., 2001]), however, we need to focus on *deep* language changes in medicine rather than word substitution, as Segal (2007) argues has happened with the concepts of *compliance* and *concordance*. Deep language change requires a systemic change of *multiple* definitions in order to move from a system that values compliance to one that values patients as partners. It is my hope is that this book can serve as a starting point for such work.

GLOSSARY

Note: Compiled from information taken from the National Institute of Diabetes and Digestive and Kidney Diseases website, Endocrineweb.com, WebMD, and the Defeat Diabetes Foundation website.

A1C: A test that provides an average blood sugar measurement over a 6- to 12-week period and is used in conjunction with home glucose monitoring to make treatment adjustments. The ideal range for people with diabetes is generally less than 7 percent. This test can also be used to diagnose diabetes.

basal rate: The amount of insulin required to manage normal daily blood glucose fluctuations; most people constantly produce insulin to manage the glucose fluctuations that occur during the day. In a person with diabetes, giving a constant low-level amount of insulin via an insulin pump mimics this normal phenomenon.

beta cell: Beta cells are located in the islets of Langerhans in the pancreas. They are responsible for making insulin.

blood glucose: This is the main sugar found in the blood and the body's main source of energy. It is also called blood sugar.

blood glucose home monitoring tests: Home glucose monitoring tests check whole blood (plasma and blood cell components); thus, the results can be different from lab values, which test plasma values of glucose. Typically, the lab plasma values tend to be higher than the glucose checks done at home with a glucose monitor.

blood glucose level: The blood glucose level is how much glucose is in a person's blood at a given time. If the blood glucose level is too high (hyperglycemia), that means that there isn't enough insulin in the blood. If it's too low (hypoglycemia), that means that there's too much insulin.

bolus: After a person eats, the pancreas releases the right amount of the hormone insulin to process the carbohydrates in the meal; that is the bolus secretion. People with type 1 diabetes must take a form of insulin that replicates the bolus secretion; that is bolus insulin.

certified diabetes educator (CDE): A health care professional who is certified by the American Association of Diabetes Educators (AADE) to teach people with diabetes how to manage their condition.

complications: The long-term effects of diabetes. They include micro- and macrovascular issues and can involve damage to the eyes; heart; blood vessels; nervous system; teeth and gums; feet and skin; or kidneys.

diabetes mellitus: A condition in which the amount of glucose (sugar) in the blood is too high because the body cannot use it properly.

diabetic ketoacidosis: Diabetic ketoacidosis (abbreviated to DKA) is a very serious condition. It occurs when there is no insulin to help the body use glucose for energy. Glucose builds up in the blood, and the body turns to fat for energy. As the body breaks down the fat, ketones are released, and when too many of those build up in the blood, it makes the blood acidic. If a person does not get immediate treatment for DKA, it can lead to a coma or death.

fasting blood glucose test: The fasting blood glucose test is one of the ways that diabetes is diagnosed. It measures the blood glucose level after fasting overnight.

gestational diabetes mellitus (GDM): A high blood sugar level that starts or is first recognized during pregnancy; hormone changes during pregnancy affect the action of insulin, resulting in high blood sugar levels. Women who have had gestational diabetes are at increased risk of developing type 2 diabetes later in life. Gestational diabetes can increase complications during labor and delivery and increase the rates of fetal complications related to the increased size of the baby.

glucose: Glucose is a major source of energy for our bodies and a building block for many carbohydrates. The food digestion process breaks down carbohydrates in foods and drinks into glucose. After digestion, glucose is carried in the blood and goes to the body's cells where it is used for energy or stored.

hyperglycemia: A a state in which there is too much glucose in the blood.

hypoglycemia: A state in which there is too little glucose in the blood.

IDDM (insulin-dependent diabetes mellitus): A former term for type 1 diabetes.

impaired fasting glucose (IFG) and impaired glucose tolerance (IGT): Conditions where glucose levels are higher than normal but not high enough to diagnose diabetes. People with IFG or IGT have an increased risk of cardiovascular disease and may go on to develop type 2 diabetes.

insulin: A hormone made by the pancreas, insulin helps move glucose (sugar) from the blood to muscles and other tissues. Insulin controls blood sugar levels.

insulin pump: A small, computerized device—about the size of a pager—that is worn on a belt or put in a pocket; insulin pumps have a small flexible tube with a fine needle on the end. The needle is inserted under the skin of the abdomen and taped in place. A carefully measured, steady flow of insulin is released into the body.

insulin resistance: When the effect of insulin on muscle, fat, and liver cells becomes less effective. This effect occurs with both insulin produced in the body and with insulin injections; therefore, higher levels of insulin are needed to lower the blood sugar.

intensive therapy/tight control: A treatment for diabetes in which blood glucose is kept as close to normal as possible. This is accomplished by frequent injections or using an insulin pump as well as diet and exercise.

islets: Groups of cells located in the pancreas that make hormones that help the body break down and use food. Also called the islets of Langerhans.

juvenile diabetes: A former term used for type 1 diabetes.

ketone: When the body starts to break down fat in order to get energy, ketones are a by-product. When too many ketones build up in the blood, it makes the blood acidic and can lead to diabetic ketoacidosis.

lancet: A fine, sharp-pointed needle for pricking the skin that is used in blood sugar monitoring.

latent autoimmune diabetes in adults (LADA): A condition in which type 1 diabetes develops in adults.

maturity-onset **diabetes of the young (MODY):** A rare type of diabetes that develops before the age of 25, runs in families, and can often be controlled by diet and physical activity alone or by activity and medication.

mg/dL: A measurement (milligrams per deciliter) that indicates the amount of a particular substance, such as glucose, in a specific amount of blood.

non-insulin-dependent **diabetes mellitus (NIDDM):** A former term for type 2 diabetes.

oral hypoglycemic agents: Medications that people take to lower the level of sugar in the blood; oral diabetes medications are prescribed for people whose pancreas still produces some insulin. Classes of these medications are alpha-glucosidase inhibitors, biguanides, D-phenylalanine derivatives, meglitinides, sulfonylureas, and thiazolidinediones.

prediabetes: Prediabetes, also called glucose intolerance, is when a person has high blood glucose levels but the levels aren't high enough *yet* to be diagnosed as diabetes. Prediabetes is an early sign of type 2 diabetes. Insulin resistance (when the body doesn't use insulin as well as it should) is another prediabetes sign.

sliding scale: A set of instructions for adjusting insulin on the basis of blood glucose test results, meals, or activity levels.

type 1 diabetes: Type 1 diabetes is thought to be an autoimmune disorder that attacks and destroys the cells in the pancreas that produce insulin. (An autoimmune disorder occurs when the body's immune system, which usually helps the body fight diseases, turns against its own tissue.) Type 1 diabetes was formerly known as "insulin-dependent diabetes mellitus," or "juvenile diabetes." Without insulin, the body is not able to use blood sugar (glucose) for energy. To treat the disease, a person must inject insulin, exercise daily, and test blood sugar several times a day.

type 2 diabetes: People with type 2 diabetes produce insulin but either their bodies do not make enough insulin or do not use the insulin they make efficiently. People with type 2 diabetes may be able to control their condition by losing weight through diet and exercise. They may also need to inject insulin or take medicine along with continuing to follow a healthy eating pattern and being physically active on a regular basis. Type 2 diabetes was formerly known as "non-insulin-dependent diabetes" or "adult-onset diabetes" and is the most common form of diabetes. Children and adolescents who are overweight may also be at risk to develop type 2 diabetes.

REFERENCES

Achter, P. (2010). Unruly bodies: The rhetorical domestication of twenty-first-century veterans of war. *Quarterly Journal of Speech, 96*(1), 46–68.

Agency for Healthcare Research and Quality (AHRQ). (2011). *Coordinating care in the medical neighborhood: Critical components and available mechanisms.* Washington, DC: U.S. Department of Health and Human Services.

Alcoff, L. M. (1988). Cultural feminism versus post-structuralism: The identity crisis in feminist theory. *Signs, 13*(3), 405–436.

American College of Physicians (ACP) (2010). *The patient-centered medical home neighbor: The interface of the patient-centered medical home with specialty/subspecialty practices.* Retrieved from https://www.acponline.org/system/files/documents/advocacy/current_policy_papers/assets/pcmh_neighbors.pdf

American Diabetes Association (ADA) (2015). Hypoglycemia (low blood sugar). Retrieved from http://www.diabetes.org/living-with-diabetes/treatment-and-care/blood-glucose-control/hypoglycemia-low-blood.html

American Diabetes Association (ADA). (2016a). *Statistics about diabetes.* Retrieved from http://www.diabetes.org/diabetes-basics/statistics/

American Diabetes Association (ADA). (2016b). Standards of medical care in diabetes-2016: Summary of revisions. *Diabetes Care, 39*(Suppl. 1), S1–S112.

Anderson, R. M., Funnell, M. M., Butler, P. M., Arnold, M. S., Fitzgerald, J. T., & Feste, C. C. (1995). Patient empowerment: Results of a randomized controlled trial. *Diabetes Care, 18*(7), 943–949.

Anderson, R. M., & Funnell, M. M. (2000). Compliance and adherence are dysfunctional concepts in diabetes care. *The Diabetes Educator, 26,* 597–604.

Anderson, R. M., & Funnell, M. M. (2010). Patient empowerment: Myths and misconceptions. *Patient Education and Counseling, 79*(3), 277–282.

Anzaldúa, G. (1983). This bridge called my back. In G. Anzaldua & C. Moraga (Eds.), *Writings by radical women of color* (pp. 252–253). Watertown, MA: Persephone.

Anzaldúa, G. (1987). *Borderlands la frontera: The new mestiza.* San Francisco, CA: AuntLuteBooks.

Applegarth, R. (2014). *Rhetoric in American anthropology: Gender, genre, and science.* Pittsburgh, PA: University of Pittsburgh Press.

Araki, M., & Carliner, S. (2008). What the literature says about using game worlds and social worlds in cyberspace for communicating technical and educational content. *Technical Communication, 55*(3), 251–260.

Arduser, L. (2011). Warp and weft: Weaving the discussion threads of an online community. *Journal of Technical Writing and Communication, 41*(1), 5–31.

Arduser, L. (2013a). Produsers and end users: How social media impacts our students' future research questions. *Communication Design Quarterly, 1*(4), 11–14.

Arduser, L. (2013b). The care and feeding of the D-beast: Metaphors of the lived experience of diabetes. In L. Meloncon (Ed.), *Rhetorical accessibility: At the intersection of technical communication and disability studies* (pp. 95–113). Amityville, NY: Baywood's Technical Communication Series.

Arduser, L. (2014). Agency in illness narratives: A pluralistic analysis. *Narrative Inquiry, 24*(1), 1–28.

Aristotle. (350 BCE). *Poetics.* The Internet Classics Archive. Retrieved from: http://classics.mit.edu/Aristotle/poetics.html

Armstrong, N., & Murphy, E. (2012). Conceptualizing resistance. *Health, 16*(3), 314–326.

Atlantis, E., Fahey, P., & Foster, J. (2014). Collaborative care for comorbid depression and diabetes: A systematic review and meta-analysis. *BMJ Open, 4*(4), 1471–1477.

Atwill, J. (1998). *Rhetoric reclaimed: Aristotle and the liberal arts tradition.* Ithaca, NY: Cornell University Press.

Auerbach, E. (2003). *Mimesis: The representation of reality in Western literature.* Princeton, NJ: Princeton University Press.

Bakhtin, M. M. (1981). *The dialogic imagination: Four essays.* Austin: University of Texas Press.

Bailey, C. J., & Kodack, M. (2011). Patient adherence to medication requirements for therapy of type 2 diabetes. *International Journal of Clinical Practice, 65*, 314–322. doi: 10.1111/j.1742-1241.2010.02544.x

Ballif, M. (1998). Writing the third-sophistic cyborg: Periphrasis on an [in]tense rhetoric. *Rhetoric Society Quarterly, 28*(4), 51–72.

Barbot, J. (2006). How to build an "active" patient? The work of AIDS associations in France. *Social Science & Medicine, 62*(3), 538–551.

Bay, J. (2010). Networking pedagogies for professional writing students. *The Writing Instructor.* Retrieved from http://files.eric.ed.gov/fulltext/EJ890608.pdf

Baynham, M. (1996). Direct speech: What's it doing in non-narrative discourse? *Journal of Pragmatics, 25*(1), 61–81.

Beer, F. (1994). Words of reason. *Political Communication, 11*(2), 185–201.

Bennett, J. A. (2009, November). *Resisting the rhetoric of diabetes 'management.'* Paper presented at the National Communication Association conference, Chicago, IL.

Bennett, J. A. (2013). Troubled interventions: Public policy, vectors of disease, and the rhetoric of diabetes management. *Journal of Medical Humanities, 34*(1), 15–32.

Berg, E. G. (2014, March). The artificial pancreas aces new tests: "Bionic" volunteers venture into the real world of ice cream and red wine. *Diabetes Forecast.* Retrieved from http://www.diabetesforecast.org/2014/mar/the-artificial-pancreas-aces.html

Berkenkotter, C. (2001). Genre systems at work: DSM-IV and rhetorical recontextualization in psychotherapy paperwork. *Written Communication, 18*(3), 326–349.

Berkenkotter, C., & Ravotas, D. (1997). Genre as tool in the transmission of practice over time and across professional boundaries. *Mind, Culture, & Activity, 4*(4), 256–274.

Berman, J. (2013). Supporter comment: Revise names of type 1 & 2 diabetes to reflect the nature of each disease. Retrieved from: https://www.change.org/p/revise-names-of-type-1-2-diabetes -to-reflect-the-nature-of-each-disease

Bhabha, H. K. (1994). *The location of culture.* New York, NY: Routledge.

Biesecker, B. A. (1989). Rethinking the rhetorical situation from within the thematic of differance. *Philosophy and Rhetoric, 22*(2), 110–130.

Biesecker, B. (1992). Michel Foucault and the question of rhetoric. *Philosophy and Rhetoric, 25*(4), 351–364.

Bitzer, L. F. (1968). The rhetorical situation. *Philosophy and Rhetoric, 1*(1), 1–14.

Bliss, M. (2007). *The discovery of insulin.* Chicago, IL: The University of Chicago Press.

Bloom, B. S. (Ed.), Engelhart, M. D., Furst, E. J., Hill, W. H., & Krathwohl, D. R. (1956). *Taxonomy of educational objectives, handbook I: The cognitive domain.* New York, NY: David McKay.

Bowker, G. C. & Star, S. L. (1999). *Sorting things out: Classification and its consequences.* Cambridge, MA: MIT Press.

Boyle, J. P., Honeycutt, A. A., Narayan, K. M., Hoerger, T. J., Geiss, L. S., Chen, H., Thompson, T. J. (2001). Projection of diabetes burden through 2050: Impact of changing demography and disease prevalence in the U. S. *Diabetes Care, 24*(11), 1936–1940.

Bragg, L. (2004). *Oedipus Borealis: The aberrant body in old Icelandic myth and saga.* Rutherford, NJ: Fairleigh Dickinson University Press.

Broom, D., & Whittaker, A. (2004). Controlling diabetes, controlling diabetics: Moral language in the management of diabetes type 2. *Social Science & Medicine, 58*(11), 2372–2382.

Brueggeman, B. J., & Voss, J. (n.d.). Articulating betweenity: Literacy, language, identity, and technology in the deaf/hard-of-hearing collection. Retrieved from http://ccdigitalpress.org/ stories/brueggemann.html

Burke, K. (1945). *A grammar of motives* Berkeley: University of California Press.

Burke, K. (1950). *A rhetoric of motives.* Berkeley: University of California Press.

Burke, K. (1966). *Language as symbolic action: Essays on life, literature and method.* Berkeley: University of California Press.

Burnett, R. E., Cooper, L. A., & Welhausen, C. A. (2013). How can technical communicators develop strategies for effective collaboration? In. J. Johnson-Eilola & S. A. Selber (Eds.), *Solving problems in technical communication* (pp. 454–478). Chicago, IL: The University of Chicago Press.

Butler, J. (1993). *Bodies that matter.* New York, NY: Routledge.

Cahn, M. (1989). Reading rhetoric rhetorically. *Rhetorica, 7,* 121–144.

Caldini, R. (1984). *Influence: The psychology of persuasion.* New York, NY: William Morrow.

Campbell, J. (2008). *The hero with a thousand faces.* Novato, CA: New World Library.

Campbell, K. K. (2005). Agency: Promiscuous and protean. *Communication and Critical/Cultural Studies, 2*(1), 1–19.

Carpman, J. R., & Grant, M. A. (2006). *Directional sense.* Boston, MA: Institute For Human Centered Design.

Centers for Disease Control and Prevention (CDC). (2016). *Chronic disease overview.* Retrieved from http://www.cdc.gov/chronicdisease/overview/

Centers for Disease Control and Prevention (CDC). (2014). *National diabetes statistics report.* Retrieved from http://www.cdc.gov/diabetes/data/statistics/2014statisticsreport.html

Centers for Disease Control (CDC). (2003). *Take charge of your diabetes.* Atlanta, GA: Department of Health and Human Services.

Cerkoney, K. A., & Hart, L. K. (1980). The relationship between the health belief model and compliance of persons with diabetes mellitus. *Diabetes Care, 3*(5), 594–598.

Charles, C., Gafni, A., & Whelan, T. (1997). Shared decision-making in the medical encounter: What does it mean? (or it takes at least two to tango). *Social Science & Medicine, 44*(5), 681–692.

Charles, C., Whelan, T., & Gafni, A. (1999). What do we mean by partnership in making decisions about treatment? *British Medical Journal, 319*(7212), 780–782.

Charon, R. (2007). What to do with stories: The sciences of narrative medicine. *Canadian Family Physician, 53*(8), 1265–1267.

Chesney, M. A., Morin, M., & Sherr, L. (2000). Adherence to HIV combination therapy. *Social Science & Medicine, 50*, 1599–1605.

Cintron, R. (1998). *Angels' town: Chero ways, gang life, and the rhetorics of everyday.* Boston, MA: Beacon Press.

Clark, H., & Gerrig, R. (1990). Quotations as demonstrations. *Language, 66*(4), 764–805.

Clarke, S. F., & Foster, J. R. (2012). A history of blood glucose meters and their role in self-monitoring of diabetes mellitus. *British Journal of Biomedical Science, 69*(2), 83–93.

Cole, K., Hall, A., Garrison, K., Ranario, M., & Tharanathan, A. (n.d.). Usability test report: Evaluation of *4 Steps to Controlling Your Diabetes for Life,* an Educational Pamphlet on Diabetes. Lubbock: Texas Tech University Usability Lab, Lubbock, TX.

Collins, H. M., & Evans, R. (2002). The third wave of science studies: Studies of expertise and experience. *Social Studies of Science, 32*(2), 235–296.

Collins, H. (2004). Interactional expertise as a third kind of knowledge. *Phenomenology and Cognitive Science, 3*(2), 125–143.

Collins, H., & Evans, R. (2007). *Rethinking expertise.* Chicago, IL: The University of Chicago Press.

Collins, J. (1923, May 6). Diabetes, dreaded disease, yields to new gland cure. *The New York Times,* p. 12.

Conrad, P. (1985). The meaning of medications: Another look at compliance. *Social Science and Medicine, 20*(1), 29–37.

Cook, C. K. (2002). Layered literacies: A theoretical frame for technical communication pedagogy. *Technical Communication Quarterly, 11*(1), 5–29.

Cooper, M. M. (2011). Rhetorical agency as emergent and enacted. *College Composition and Communication, 62*(3), 420–449.

Corbett, E. P. J. (1971). The theory and practice of imitation in classical rhetoric. *College Composition and Communication, 22*(3), 243–250.

Corbin, J. M., & Strauss, A. (1988). *Unending work and care: Managing chronic illness at home.* San Francisco, CA: Jossey-Bass Publishers.

Crampton, J. N., & Elden, S. (Eds.). (2007). *Space, knowledge and power: Foucault and geography.* London, UK: Ashgate.

Crowley, S. (1985). Rhetoric, literature, and the dissociation of invention. *Journal of Advanced Composition, 6*, 17–32.

Deardorff, J. (2010, November 22). Diabetes' civil war: People with type 1 diabetes, outnumbered and overshadowed by type 2, fight for recognition, resources—and a new name for their disorder. *The Chicago Tribune.* Retrieved from http://articles.chicagotribune.com/2010-11-22/a-z/ct-met-diabetes-rift-20101122_1_diabetes-insulin-lifestyle-changes-and-medication

de Certeau, M. (1984). *The practice of everyday life.* Berkeley: University of California Press.

Deleuze, G., & Guattari, F. (1981). Rhizome. *Ideology & Consciousness, 8*, 49–71.

Deleuze, G., & Guattari, F. (1987). *A thousand plateaus: Capitalism and schizophrenia.* Minneapolis, MN: University of Minnesota Press.

DeLuca, K. (1999). Articulation theory: A discursive grounding for rhetorical practice. *Philosophy and Rhetoric, 32*(4), 334–348.

Derkatch, C., & Segal, J. Z. (2005). Realms of rhetoric in health and medicine. *University of Toronto Medical Journal, 82*(2), 138–142.

de Swaan, A. (1981). The politics of agoraphobia: On changes in emotional and relational management. *Theory and Society, 10*(3), 359–385.

Detienne, M., & Vernant, J. (1978). *Cunning intelligence in Greek culture and society.* Chicago, IL: The University of Chicago Press.

Diabetes Control and Complications Trial (DCCT) Group. (1993). The effect of intensive treatment of diabetes on the development and progression of long-term complications in insulin-dependent diabetes mellitus. *New England Journal of Medicine, 329*(14), 977–986.

Doheny-Farina, S. (2004). Writing in an emerging organization: An ethnographic study. In J. Johnson-Eilola & S. A. Selber (Eds.), *Central works in technical communication* (pp. 325–340). New York, NY: Oxford University Press.

Dolmage, J. (2009). Metis, metis, mestiza, Medusa: Rhetorical bodies across rhetorical traditions. *Rhetoric Review, 28*(1), 1–28.

Douglas, M. (1992). *Risk and blame: Essays in cultural theory.* New York, NY: Routledge.

Duin, A. H., & Hansen, C. J. (1996). *Nonacademic writing: Social theory and technology.* Mahweh, NJ: Lawrence Erlbaum Associates.

Dunne, J. (1993). *Back to the rough ground: Practical judgment and the lure of technique.* Notre Dame, IN: University of Notre Dame Press.

Edbauer, J. (2005). Unframing models of public distribution: From rhetorical situation to rhetorical ecologies. *Rhetoric Society Quarterly, 35*(4), 5–24.

Eldredge, N., & Gould, S. J. (1972). Punctuated equilibria: An alternative to phyletic gradualism. In T. J. M. Schopf (Ed.), *Models in paleobiology* (pp. 82–115). San Francisco, CA: Freeman Cooper.

Emmons, K. K. (2010). *Black dogs and blue words: Depression and gender in the age of self-care.* New Brunswick, NJ: Rutgers University Press.

Enck-Wanzer, D. (2011). Tropicalizing East Harlem: Rhetorical agency, cultural citizenship, and Nuyorican cultural production. *Communication Theory, 21*(4), 344–367.

Epstein, S. (2000). Democracy, expertise, and AIDS treatment activism. In D. Kleinman (Ed.), *Science, technology, and democracy* (pp. 15–32). Albany: State University of New York Press.

Fahnestock, J. (1986). Accommodating science: The rhetorical life of scientific facts. *Written Communication, 3*(3), 275–296.

Ferguson, K. L. (2010). The cinema of control: On diabetic excess and illness in film. *Journal of Medical Humanities, 31*(3), 183–204.

Feudtner, C. (2003). *Bittersweet: Diabetes, insulin, and the transformation of illness.* Chapel Hill: The University of North Carolina Press.

Fisher, E. S. (2008). Building a medical neighborhood for the medical home. *New England Journal of Medicine, 359*(12), 1202–1205.

Foucault, M. (1977). What is an author? In D. F. Bouchard (Ed.), *Language, counter-memory, practice* (pp. 124–127). Ithaca, NY: Cornell University Press.

Foucault, M. (1980). *Power/knowledge: Selected interviews and other writings, 1972–1977.* New York, NY: Pantheon Books.

Foucault, M. (1983). Afterword: The subject of power. In H. L. Dreyfus & P. Rabinow (Eds.), *Michel Foucault: Beyond structuralism and hermeneutics* (pp. 208–228). Chicago: University of Chicago Press.

Foucault, M. (1984a). Of other spaces, heterotopias. *Architecture, Mouvement, Continuité, 5,* 46–49.

Foucault, M. (1984b). What is an author? In P. Rabinow (Ed.), *The Foucault reader* (pp. 101–120). New York, NY: Pantheon Books.

Foucault, M. (1994). *The birth of the clinic: An archaeology of medical perception.* New York, NY: Vintage Books.

Fountain, T. K. (2014). *Rhetoric in the Flesh: Trained vision, technical expertise, and the gross anatomy lab.* New York, NY: Routledge.

Freire, P. (1993). *Pedagogy of the oppressed.* New York, NY: Continuum.

Gebel, E. (2010, May). The other diabetes: LADA, or type 1.5 *Diabetes Forecast.* Retrieved from http://www.diabetesforecast.org

Geisler, C. (2004). How ought we understand the concept of rhetorical agency? Report from the ARS. *Rhetoric Society Quarterly, 34*(3), 9–17.

Glasgow, R. E., & Anderson, R. M. (1999). In diabetes care, moving from compliance to adherence is not enough. *Diabetes Care, 22*(12), 2090–2092.

Goodnight, G. T., & Green, S. (2010). Rhetoric, risk, and the markets: The dot com bubble. *Quarterly Journal of Speech, 96*(2), 115–140.

Gorsevski, E. W., Schuck, R. I., & Lin, C. (2012). The rhetorical plasticity of the dead in museum displays: A biocritique of missing intercultural awareness. *Western Journal of Communication, 76*(3), 314–332.

Grabill, J. T., & Pigg, S. (2012). Messy rhetoric: Identity performance as rhetorical agency in online public forums. *Rhetoric Society Quarterly, 42*(2), 99–119.

Grabill, J. T., & Simmons, M. W. (1998). Toward a critical rhetoric of risk communication: Producing citizens and the role of technical communicators. *Technical Communication Quarterly, 7,* 415–441.

Graham, S. (2009). Agency and the rhetoric of medicine: Biomedical brain scans and the ontology of fibromyalgia. *Technical Communication Quarterly, 18*(4), 376–404.

Gramsci, A. (1971). *Selections from the prison notebooks* (Q. Hoare & G. Smith, Trans.) London, UK: Lawrence & Wishart.

Greene, J. A., Choudhry, N. K., Kilabuk, E., & Shrank, W. H. (2011). Online social networking by patients with diabetes: A qualitative evaluation of communication with Facebook. *Journal of General Internal Medicine, 26*(3), 287–292.

Greene, R. W. (1998). Another materialist rhetoric. *Critical Studies in Media Communication, 15*(1), 21–40.

Greene, R. W. (2004). Rhetoric and capitalism: Rhetorical agency as communicative labor. *Philosophy and Rhetoric, 37*(3), 188–206.

Gries, L. (2012). Agential matters: Tumbleweed, women-pens, citizen-hope, and rhetorical actancy. In S. J. Dobrin (Ed.), *Ecology, writing theory, and new media* (pp. 67–91). New York, NY: Routledge.

Grossberg, L. (1987). Critical theory and the politics of empirical research. In M. Glirevitch & M. R. Levy (Eds.), *Mass Communication Review Yearbook* (pp. 86–106). London, UK: Sage.

Grossberg, L. (1989). The circulation of cultural studies. *Critical Studies in Mass Communication, 6,* 413–421.

Grossberg, L. (1993). Cultural studies and/in new worlds. *Critical Studies in Mass Communication, 10,* 1–22.

Grosz, E. (1994). *Volatile bodies: Toward a corporeal feminism.* Bloomington: Indiana University Press.

Grove, L. K., Lundgren, R. E., & Hays, F. C. (1992). Winning respect throughout the organization. *Technical Communication, 41,* 424–431.

Grundy, S. M. (2012). Pre-diabetes, metabolic syndrome, and cardiovascular risk. *Journal of the American College of Cardiology, 59*(7), 635–643.

Hak, T., & de Boer, F. (1996). Formulations in first encounters. *Journal of Pragmatics, 25*(1), 83–99.

Hall, S. (1985). Signification, representation, ideology: Althusser and the post-structuralist debates. *Critical Studies in Mass Communication, 2*(2), 91–114.

Hall, S. (1986). On postmodernism and articulation: An interview with Stuart Hall. *Journal of Communication Inquiry, 10*(2), 45–60.

Hall, S. (2000). "Who needs 'identity'?" In P. du Gay, J. Evans, & P. Redman (Eds.), *Identity: A reader* (pp. 15–30). London: Sage Publications Ltd.

Hall, S. (2001). Foucault: Power, knowledge and discourse. In M. Wetherell, S. Taylor, & S. J. Yates (Eds.), *Discourse theory and practice: A reader* (pp. 72–80). Thousand Oaks, CA: Sage.

Hallenbeck, S. (2012). User agency, technical communication, and the nineteenth-century woman bicyclist. *Technical Communication Quarterly, 21*(4), 290–306.

Hanne, M., & Hawken, S. J. (2007). Metaphors for illness in contemporary media. *Medical Humanities, 33*(2), 93–99.

Hanselman, S. (2014, June 30). Diabetics: It's fun to say bionic pancreas but how about a reality check. *Scott Hanselman.* Retrieved from http://www.hanselman.com/blog/DiabeticsItsFunToSayBionicPancreasButHowAboutARealityCheck.aspx

Haraway, D. (1991). *Simians, cyborgs and women: The reinvention of nature.* New York, NY: Routledge.

Haraway, D. (1992). The promises of monsters: A Regenerative politics for inappropriate/d others. In L. Grossberg, C. Nelson, & P. A. Treichler (Eds.), *Cultural studies* (pp. 295–337). New York, NY: Routledge.

Harding, S. G. (1991). *Whose science? Whose knowledge?: Thinking from women's lives.* Ithaca, NY: Cornell University Press.

Harris, R., & Linn, M. W. (1985). Health beliefs, compliance, and control of diabetes mellitus. *Southern Medical Journal, 78*(2), 162–166.

Hartelius, E. J. (2011). *The rhetoric of expertise*. Lanham, MD: Lexington Books.

Harvey, R. (1998). The judgement of urines. *Canadian Medical Association Journal, 159*(12), 1482–1484.

Hauser, G. A., & Kjeldsen, J. E. (2010). Rhetorical situations in everyday discourse. In J. Kangira & P. J. Salazar (Eds.), *Gender rhetoric: North-South* (pp. 91–100). Windhoek, Namibia: Poly Press Namibia.

Heaton, J., Räisänen, U., & Salinas, M. (2016). 'Rule your condition, don't let it rule you': Young adults' sense of mastery in their accounts of growing up with a chronic illness. *Sociology of Health & Illness, 38*(1), 3–20. doi:10.1111/1467-9566.12298

Heid, V. (2006). *The ethics of care: Personal, political, and global*. New York, NY: Oxford University Press.

Hengst, J. A., Frame, S. R., Neuman-Stritzel, T., & Gannaway, R. (2005). Using others' words: Conversational use of reported speech by individuals with aphasia and their communication partners. *Journal of Speech, Language, and Hearing Research, 48*(1), 137–156.

Henry, J. (1994). Toward technical authorship. *Journal of Technical Writing and Communication, 24*(4), 449–461.

Henry, J. (1998). Documenting contributory expertise. *Technical Communication. 45*(2), 207–220.

Henry, J. (2000). *Writing workplace cultures: An archaeology of professional writing*. Carbondale: Southern Illinois University Press.

Herndl, C. G., & Licona, A. C. (2007). Shifting agency: Agency, kairos, and the possibilities of social action. In M. Zachary & C. Thralls (Eds.), *Communicative practices in workplaces and the professions: Cultural perspectives on the regulation of discourse and organizations* (pp. 133–153). Amityville, NY: Baywood.

Herzlich, C., & Pierret, J. (1987). *Illness and self in society*. Baltimore, MD: Johns Hopkins University Press.

Hetherington, K. (1997). *The badlands of modernity: Heterotopia and social ordering,* New York, NY: Routledge.

Hill, I. (2009). "The human barnyard" and Kenneth Burke's philosophy of technology. *The Journal of the Kenneth Burke Society, 5*(2). Retrieved from http://www.kbjournal.org/ian_hill

hooks, b. (2000). *Feminism is for everybody: Passionate politics*. London, UK: Pluto Press.

Horvath, A. (2013). *Modernism and charisma*. Houndmills, UK: Palgrave Macmillan.

Howard, T. (2014). Journey mapping: A brief overview. *Communication Design Quarterly, 2*(3), 10–13.

Howard-Thompson, A., Farland, M. Z., Byrd, D. C., Airee, A., Thomas, J., Campbell, J., Cassidy, R., Morgan, T., & Suda, K. J. (2013). Pharmacist-physician collaboration for diabetes care: Cardiovascular outcomes. *Annals of Pharmacotherapy, 47*(11), 1471–1477.

Hubbard, P., Kitchin, R., & Valentine, G. (Eds). (2004). *Key thinkers on space and place*. London, UK: Sage.

Hyland, K. (1996). Writing without conviction? Hedging in science research articles. *Applied Linguistics, 17*(4), 433–454.

Hyland, K. (2000). *Disciplinary discourse: Social interactions in academic writing*. Harlow, UK: Longman.

Improving Chronic Illness Care. (2016). The Chronic Care Model. Retrieved from http://www.improvingchroniccare.org/index.php?p=The_Chronic_Care_Model&s=2

Institute of Medicine. (2001a). Crossing the quality chasm: A new health system for the 21st century. Washington, DC: National Academies Press.

Institute of Medicine. (2001b). Envisioning the National Health Care Quality Report. Washington, DC: National Academies Press.

International Diabetes Federation (IDF). (2015). Who we are. *International Diabetes Federation.* Retrieved from: http://www.idf.org/who-we-are

International Expert Committee. (2009). International Expert Committee report on the role of the A1C assay in the diagnosis of diabetes. *Diabetes Care, 32*(7), 1327–1334.

Jaggar, A. (1991). Feminist ethics: Problems, projects, prospects. In C. Card (Ed.), *Feminist ethics* (pp. 78–104). Lawrence: University Press of Kansas.

Jasinski, J. (2001). *Sourcebook on rhetoric: Key concepts in contemporary rhetorical studies.* Thousand Oaks, CA: Sage.

Jeyaraj, J. (2004). Liminality and othering: The issue of rhetorical authority in technical discourse. *Journal of Business and Technical Communication, 18*(1), 9–38.

Johnson, J. A., Al Sayah, F., Wozniak, L., Rees, S., Soprovich, A., Qiu, W., Chik, C. L., Chue, P., Florence, P., Jacquier, J., Lysak, P., Opgenorth, A., Katon, W., & Majumdar, S. R. (2014). Collaborative care versus screening and follow-up for patients with diabetes and depressive symptoms: Results of a primary care-based comparative effectiveness trial. *Diabetes Care, 37*(12), 3220–3226.

Johnson, R. R. (1997). Audience involved: Toward a participatory model of writing. *Computers and Composition, 14*(3), 361–376.

Johnson, R. R. (1998). *User-centered technology: A rhetorical theory for computers and other mundane artifacts.* Albany: State University of New York Press.

Johnson-Eilola, J. (1996). Relocating the value of work: Technical communication in a post-industrial age. *Technical Communication Quarterly, 5*(3), 245–270.

Johnson-Eilola, J. (2005). *Datacloud: Toward a new theory of online work.* Cresskill, NJ: Hampton Press.

Johnson-Eilola, J., & Selber, S. A. (Eds.). (2004). *Central works in technical communication.* New York, NY: Oxford University Press

Johnson-Eilola, J., & Selber, S. A. (Eds.). (2013). *Solving problems in technical communication.* Chicago: The University of Chicago Press.

Jordan, J. W. (2004). The rhetorical limits of the "plastic body." *Quarterly Journal of Speech, 90*(3), 327–358.

Jordan, J. W. (2009). Reshaping the "pillow angel": Plastic bodies and the rhetoric of normal surgical solutions. *Quarterly Journal of Speech, 95*(1), 20–42.

Juvenile Diabetes Research Foundation (JDRF). (2016). About JDRF. *JDRF.org.* Retrieved from http://www.jdrf.org/about/

Keränen, L. (2007). 'Cause someday we all die: Rhetoric, agency, and the case of the patient preferences worksheet. *Quarterly Journal of Speech, 93*(2), 179–210.

Kerber, L. K. (1988). Separate spheres, female worlds, woman's place: The rhetoric of women's history. *The Journal of American History, 75*(1), 9–39.

Kimball, M. (2006). Cars, culture, and tactical technical communication. *Technical Communication Quarterly, 15*(1), 67–86.

Koerber, A. (2006). Rhetorical agency, resistance, and the disciplinary rhetorics of breastfeeding. *Technical Communication Quarterly, 15*(1), 87–101.

Koerber, A. (2013). *Breast or bottle? Contemporary controversies in infant-feeding policy and practice.* Columbia: The University of South Carolina Press.

Kopelson, K. (2003). Rhetoric on the edge of cunning; or, the performance of neutrality (re)considered as a composition pedagogy for student resistance. *College Composition and Communication, 55*(1), 115–146.

Kuhn, T. S. (1962). *The structure of scientific revolutions.* Chicago, IL: The University of Chicago Press.

Laclau, E. (1977). *Politics and ideology in Marxist theory.* London, UK: Verso.

Lakoff, G., & Johnson, M. (1980). *Metaphors we live by.* Chicago, IL: The University of Chicago Press.

Lakshmanan, I. (Host). (2016, February 9). Improving doctor-patient communication in a digital world [Radio broadcast episode]. In S. Casey (Producer), *The Diane Rehm Show.* Washington, DC: National Public Radio.

Lancet. (2009). Tackling the burden of chronic diseases in the USA. *Lancet, 373*(9659), 185. Retrieved from http://thelancet.com/journals/lancet/article/PIIS0140-6736(09)60048-9/fulltext

Latour, B. (1987). *Science in action: How to follow scientists and engineers through society.* Cambridge, MA: Harvard University Press.

Latour, B. (1993). *We have never been modern.* Cambridge, MA: Harvard University Press.

Latour, B. (1999). Pandora's hope: Essays on the reality of science studies. Cambridge, MA: Harvard University Press.

Law, J. (2002). Objects and spaces. *Theory, Culture & Society, 19*(5–6), 91–105.

Lay, M. M. (2000). *The rhetoric of midwifery: Gender, knowledge and power.* New Brunswick, NJ: Rutgers University Press.

Lefebvre, H. (1991). *The production of space.* (D. Nicholson-Smith, Trans.). Malden, MA: Blackwell Publishing. (Original work published 1974.)

Leff, M. (1997). Hermeneutical rhetoric. In W. Jost & M. J. Hyde (Eds.), *Rhetoric and hermeneutics in our time: A reader* (pp. 196–214). New Haven, CT: Yale University Press.

Leff, M. (2003). Tradition and agency in humanistic rhetoric. *Philosophy and Rhetoric, 36*(2), 135–147.

Leslie. (2008, August 28). Predictably unpredictable. [Blog comment]. *Type1Parents.* Retrieved from http://type1parents.org

Lewiecki-Wilson, C., & Cellio, J. (Eds.). (2011). *Disability and mothering: Liminal spaces of embodied knowledge.* Syracuse, NY: Syracuse University Press.

Lillie, E. O., Patay, B., Diamant, J., Issell, B., Topol, E. J., & Schork, N. J. (2011). The n-of-1 clinical trial: The ultimate strategy for individualizing medicine? *Perspectives in Medicine, 8*(2), 161–173.

Linton, S. (1998). *Claiming disability: Knowledge and identity.* New York: New York University Press.

Lupton, D. (1995). *The imperative of health: Public health and the regulated body.* London, UK: Sage.

Lupton, D. (2003). *Medicine as culture.* London, UK: Sage.

Lupton, D. (2013). *Risk*. London, UK: Routledge.

Lynch, J. (2009). New agendas in science communication. In L. Kahlor & P. Stout (Eds.), *Exemplary creatures: Articulation and the organization of scientific materiality, sociality and rhetoric* (pp. 161–186). New York, NY: Lawrence Erlbaum Associates.

Lynch, J. (2011). *What are stem cells? Definitions at the intersection of science and politics*. Tuscaloosa: The University of Alabama Press.

MacDonald, S. P. (2005). The language of journalism in treatments of hormone replacement news. *Written Communication, 22*(3), 275–297.

Mackenzie, C., & Stoljar, N. (Eds.). (2000). Relational autonomy: Feminist perspectives on autonomy, agency, and the social self. New York, NY: Oxford University Press.

Mackiewicz, J. (2010). Assertions of expertise in online product reviews. *Journal of Business and Technical Communication, 24*(1), 3–28.

Malmsheimer, R. (1988). *Doctors only: The evolving image of the American physician*. Westport, CT: Greenwood Press.

Mansfield, N. (2000). *Subjectivity: Theories of the self from Freud to Haraway*. New York: New York University Press.

Martins, D. S. (2005). Compliance rhetoric and the impoverishment of context. *Communication Theory, 15*(1), 59–77.

Martins, D. S. (2009). Diabetes and literacy: Negotiating control through artifacts of medicalization. *Journal of Medical Humanities, 30*(2), 115–130.

Masley, S., Sokoloff, J., & Hawes, C. (2000). Planning group visits for high risk patients. *Family Practice Management, 7*(6), 1–7.

Maslow, A. H. (2015). *A theory of human motivation*. Boise, ID: Rediscovered Books.

McCarthy, L. P. (1991). A psychiatrist using DSM-III: The influence of a charter document in psychiatry. In C. Bazerman & J. Paradis (Eds.), *Textual dynamics of the professions: Historical and contemporary studies of writing in professional communities* (pp. 358–378). Madison: University of Wisconsin Press.

McCarthy, L. P., & Gerring, J. P. (1994). Revisiting psychiatry's charter document DSM-IV. *Written Communication, 11*(2), 147–192.

McCarthy, M. (2010, February 13). Harvard Vanguard finds success with unusual model of group appointments. *The Patriot Ledger*. Retrieved from http://www.patriotledger.com/

McInaney, M. (2000, October 18). Group appointments can benefit busy doctors and chronically ill patients, according to UCSF research. *University of California San Francisco (UCSF) News Center*. Retrieved from http://news.ucsf.edu

McKeon, R. (1936). Literary criticism and the concept of imitation in antiquity. *Modern Philology, 34*(1), 1–35.

McNely, B. (2014). Knowledge work, knowledge play: A heuristic approach to communication design for hybrid spaces. *Communication Design Quarterly, 2*(4), 14–51.

Mehl-Madrona, L. (2010). Comparisons of health education, group medical care, and collaborative health care for controlling diabetes. *The Permanente Journal, 14*(2), 4–10.

Melberg, A. (1995). *Theories of mimesis*. Cambridge, MA: Cambridge University Press.

Metcalf, E. (2008, April 11). My doctor treated me like a child. *Health*. Retrieved from http://www.health.com/health/condition-article/0,,20191002,00.html

Miller, C. R. (1984). Genre as social action. *Quarterly Journal of Speech, 70*, 151–167.

Miller, C. R. (1989a). What's practical about technical writing?" In B. E. Fearing & W. K. Sparrow (Eds.), *Technical writing: Theory and practice* (pp. 14–24). New York: Modern Language Association.

Miller, C. R. (1989b). The rhetoric of decision science, or Herbert A. Simon says. *Science, Technology, & Human Values, 14*(1), 43–46.

Miller, C. R. (2000). The Aristotelian topos: Hunting for novelty. In A. G. Gross & A. E. Walzer (Eds.), *Rereading Aristotle's rhetoric* (pp. 130–146). Carbondale: Southern Illinois University Press.

Miller, C. R. (2004). Expertise and agency: Transformations of ethos in human-computer interaction. In M. Hyde (Ed.), *The ethos of rhetoric* (pp. 197–218). Columbia: University of South Carolina Press.

Miller, C. R. (2007). What can automation tell us about agency? *Rhetoric Society Quarterly, 37*(2), 137–157.

Miller, C. R., & Shepherd, D. (2004). Blogging as social action: A genre analysis of the weblog. In L. Gurak, S. Antonijevic, L. Johnson, C. Ratliff, and J. Reyman (Eds.), *Into the Blogosphere: Rhetoric, Community, and Culture of Weblogs*. Minneapolis, MN: University of Minnesota Libraries.

Miller, C. R., & Shepherd, D. (2009). Questions for genre theory from the blogosphere. In J. Giltrow & D. Stein (Eds.), *Genres in the Internet* (pp. 263–290). Amsterdam, Neth.: John Benjamins Publishing Company.

Miller, L. G., & Hays, R. D. (2000). Adherence to combination antiretroviral therapy: Synthesis of the literature and clinical implications. *The AIDS Reader, 10*, 177–185.

Mishler, E. G. (1984). *The discourse of medicine: Dialectics of the medical interview*. Norwood, NJ: Ablex.

Moeller, R. M., & McAllister, K. S. (2002). Playing with techne: A propaedeutic for technical communications. *Technical Communication Quarterly, 11*(2), 185–206.

Mol, A. (2002). *The body multiple: Ontology in medical practice*. Durham, NC: Duke University Press.

Mol, A. (2008). *The logic of care: Health and the problem of patient choice*. London, UK: Routledge.

Mol, A., & Law, J. (2004). Embodied action, enacted bodies: The example of hypoglycaemia. *Body & Society, 10*(2–3), 43–62.

Montori, V. M., Gafni, A., & Charles, C. (2006). A shared treatment decision-making approach between patients with chronic conditions and their clinicians: The case of diabetes. *Health Expectations, 9*(1), 25–36.

Mountford, R. (2001). On gender and rhetorical space. *Rhetoric Society Quarterly, 31*(1), 41–71.

Mykhalovskiy, E., McCoy, L., & Bresalier, M. (2004). Compliance/adherence, HIV, and the critique of medical power. *Social Theory & Health, 2*(4), 315–340.

Naemiratch, B., & Manderson, L. (2006). Control and adherence: Living with diabetes in Bangkok, Thailand. *Social Science & Medicine, 63*, 1147–1157.

National Diabetes Data Group (NDDG). (1979). Classification and diagnosis of diabetes mellitus and other categories of glucose intolerance. *Diabetes, 28*(12), 1039–1057.

National Institute of Diabetes and Digestive and Kidney Diseases (NIDDK). (2015). *National diabetes education program*. Retrieved from http://www.niddk.nih.gov

National Institutes of Health (NIH). (2014). About grants. *NIH*. Retrieved from: http://grants.nih.gov/grants/about_grants.htm

National Institutes of Health (NIH). (2016, February 23)."Invisible work" toll among family and unpaid caregivers. *NIH Research Matters*. Retrieved from https://www.nih.gov/news-events/nih-research-matters/invisible-work-toll-among-family-unpaid-caregivers

Neuberger, J, (1999). Let's do away with "patients." *BMJ Open, 318*(7200), 1756–1758.

New Media Consortium and EDUCAUSE Learning Initiative. (2007). *The horizon report.* Retrieved from http://www.nmc.org/pdf/2007_Horizon_Report.pdf

The New York Times. (1915, August 22). Senator Shively very ill: Indiana representative suffers from a septic form of diabetes. *The New York Times*, p. 13. ProQuest Historical Newspapers.

The New York Times. (1922, December 22). Tells of diabetes cure. Dr. Banting lectures on insulin before the Academy of Medicine. *The New York Times*, p. 9. ProQuest Historical Newspapers.

The New York Times. (1935, July 3). Urge more use of insulin: Experts find that fear now blocks the cure of diabetes. *The New York Times*, p. 15. ProQuest Historical Newspapers.

The New York Times. (1956, February 19). New drug treats breast cancer. *The New York Times*, p. 65. ProQuest Historical Newspapers.

Noffsinger, E., & Scott, J. (2000). Understanding today's group visit models. *The Permanente Journal, 4*(2), 1–29.

Oliveirai, R. F. (2009). Social behavior in context: Hormonal modulation of behavioral plasticity and social competence. *Integrative & Comparative Biology, 49*(4), 423–440.

Owens, K. H. (2009). Confronting rhetorical disability: A critical analysis of women's birth plans. *Written Communication, 26*(3), 247–272.

Papillion, T. (1995). Isocrates' techne and rhetorical pedagogy. *Rhetoric Society Quarterly, 25*(1–4), 149–163.

Parsons, T. (1951). *The social system.* New York, NY: Free Press.

Patient-Centered Outcomes Research Institute (PCORI). (2014). About us. *pcori.org*. Retrieved from http://www.pcori.org/about-us

Peel, E., Parry, O., Douglas, M., & Lawton, J. (2005). Taking the biscuit? A discursive approach to managing diet in type 2 diabetes. *Journal of Health Psychology, 10*, 779–791.

Pendry, D. A. (2003). *Control, compliance, and common sense power relations in diabetes care for Mexican Americans* (Doctoral dissertation, The University of Texas, Austin). Retrieved from https://www.lib.utexas.edu/etd/d/2003/pendrydao32/pendrydao32.pdf

Perleman, C., & Olbrechts, L. (1969). *The new rhetoric.* Notre Dame, IN: University of Notre Dame Press.

Persson, A., & Richards, W. (2008). From closet to heterotopia: A conceptual exploration of disclosure and 'passing' among heterosexuals living with HIV. *Culture, Health and Sexuality, 10*(1), 73–86.

Petty, T. (2015). A statement from Tom Petty. *TomPetty.com*. Retrieved from http://www.tompetty.com/blog/statement-tom-petty-422041

Pham, H. H. (2010). Good neighbors: How will the patient-centered medical home relate to the rest of the health care delivery system? *Journal of General Internal Medicine, 25*(6), 630–634.

Phelps, L. W. (1988). *Composition as a human science.* New York, NY: Oxford University Press.

Phillips, K. R. (2006). Rhetorical maneuvers: Subjectivity, power, and resistance. *Philosophy and Rhetoric, 39*(4), 310–332.

Pomerantz, A., & Rintel, E. S. (2004). Practices for reporting and responding to test results during medical consultations: Enacting the roles of paternalism and independent expertise. *Discourse Studies, 6*(1), 9–26.

Popham, S. L. (2005). Forms as boundary genres in medicine, science, and business. *Journal of Business and Technical Communication, 19*(3), 279–303.

Popham, S. L. (2014). Hybrid disciplinarity: Métis and ethos in juvenile mental health electronic records. *Journal of Technical Writing and Communication, 44*(3), 329–344.

Popham, S. L., & Graham, S. L. (2008). A structural analysis of coherence in electronic charts in juvenile mental health. *Technical Communication Quarterly, 17*(2), 149–172.

Porter, R. (1999). *The greatest benefit to mankind: A medical history of humanity.* New York, NY: W. W. Norton & Company.

Purcell, K., & Rainie, L. (2014). More information yields more learning and sharing. Retrieved from http://www.pewinternet.org/2014/12/08/more-information-yields-more-learning-and -sharing/

Quick, C. (2012). From the workplace to academia: Nontraditional students and the relevance of workplace experience in technical writing pedagogy. *Technical Communication Quarterly, 21*(3), 230–250.

Radcliffe, J. (2014). Joining the Rapid7 team! Rapid7community. Retrieved from: https://community .rapid7.com/community/rapid7-news/blog/authors/jradcliffe

Ravotas, D., & Berkenkotter, C. (1998). Voices in the text: The uses of reported speech in a psychotherapist's notes and initial assessments. *Text—Interdisciplinary Journal for the Study of Discourse, 18*, 211–240.

Rawlins, J. D., & Wilson, G. D. (2014). Agency and interactive data displays: Internet graphics as co-created rhetorical spaces. *Technical Communication Quarterly, 23*, 303–322.

Reich, R. B. (1991). *The work of nations: Preparing ourselves for 21st century capitalism.* New York, NY: Alfred A. Knopf.

Reuters. (2014, May 29). Rapid7 hires Jay Radcliffe, diabetic who hacked his insulin pump. *Reuters.* Retrieved from http://www.reuters.com/article/us-rapid7-radcliffe -idUSKBN0E929K20140529

Rice, D., & Sweeney, K. (2013, April 17). Choosing and using an insulin pump infusion set. *Diabetes Self-Management.* Retrieved from http://www.diabetesselfmanagement.com/diabetes -resources/tools-tech/choosing-and-using-an-insulin-pump-infusion-set/

Rock, M. (2005). Classifying diabetes; or, commensurating bodies of unequal experience. *Public Culture, 17*(3), 467–486.

Roochnik, D. (1996). *Of art and wisdom: Plato's understanding of technê.* University Park: Pennsylvania State University Press.

Rosenhek, J. (2005). Liquid gold. *Doctor's Review: Medicine on the move.* Retrieved from http:// www.doctorsreview.com/history/sep05_history/

Ruggiero, L., Moadsiri, A., Quinn, L. T., Riley, B. B., Danielson, K. K., Monahan, C., Bangs, V. A., & Gerber, B. S. (2014). Diabetes island: Preliminary impact of a virtual world self-care educational intervention for African Americans with type 2 diabetes. *Journal of Medical Internet Research Serious Games, 2*(2), e10.

Saaddine, J. B., Engelgau, M. M., Beckles, G. L., Gregg, E. W., Thompson, T. J., & Narayan, K. M. (2002). A diabetes report card for the United States: Quality of care in the 1990s. *Annals of Internal Medicine, 136*(8), 565–574.

Safford, M. M., Russell, L., Suh, D., Roman, S., & Pogach, L. (2005). How much time do patients with diabetes spend on self care? *Journal of the American Board of Family Medicine, 18*(4), 262–270.

Sahlins, M. D., & Service, E. R. (Eds). (1960). *Evolution and Culture.* Ann Arbor, MI: University of Michigan Press.

Salvo, M. J. (2006). Rhetoric as productive technology: Cultural studies in/as technical communication methodology. In J. B. Scott, B. Longo, & K. V. Wills (Eds.), *Critical power tools: Technical communication and cultural studies* (pp. 219–240). Albany: State University of New York Press.

Sandison, S. (2014). Defeating diabetes. *Miss Idaho.* Retrieved from http://missidahoorg.blogspot .com

Sanger-Katz, M., & Cox, A. (2014, September 17). With new health law, shopping around can be crucial. Retrieved from http://www.nytimes.com/2014/09/18/upshot/with-new-health-law -shopping-around-can-be-crucial.html

Sauer, B. J. (2003). *The rhetoric of risk: Technical documentation in hazardous environments.* Mahwah, NJ: Lawrence Erlbaum Associates.

Schryer, C. F. (1993). Records as genres. *Written Communication, 10*(2), 200–234.

Schryer, C. F. (1994). The lab vs. the clinic: Sites of competing genres. In A. Freedman & P. Medway (Eds.), *Genre and the new rhetoric* (pp. 105–124). London, UK: Taylor and Francis.

Schryer, C. F., Bell, S., Mian, M., Spafford, M. M., & Lingard, L. (2011). Professional citation practices in child maltreatment forensic letters. *Written Communication, 28*(2), 147–171.

Schryer, C. F., Campbell, S. L., Spafford, M. M., & Lingard, L. (2006). You are how you cite: Citing patient information in health care settings. In A. Freedman & N. Artemeva (Eds.), *Rhetorical genre studies and beyond* (pp. 143–137).Winnipeg, Manitoba, Canada: Inkshed Press.

Schryer, C. F., Lingard, L., & Spafford, M. M. (2005). Techne or artful science and the genre of case presentations in healthcare settings. *Communication Monographs, 72*(2), 234–260.

Schryer, C. F., Lingard, L., Spafford, M. M., & Garwood, K. (2003). Structure and agency in medical case presentations. In D. Russell (Ed.), *Writing selves/writing societies: Research from activity perspectives* (pp. 63–96). Fort Collins, CO: The WAC Clearinghouse. Retrieved from: http://wac.colostate.edu/books/selves_societies/schryer/.

Schryer, C. F., & Spoel, P. (2005). Genre theory, healthcare discourse, and professional identity formation. *Journal of Business and Technical Communication, 19*(3), 249–278.

Scott, J. B. (2003). *Risky rhetoric: AIDS and the cultural practice of HIV testing.* Carbondale: Southern Illinois University Press.

Scott, J. B., Longo, B., & Wills, K. V. (Eds.). (2006). *Critical power tools: Technical communication and cultural studies.* Albany: State University of New York Press.

Scott, J. B., Segal, J. Z., & Keränen, L. (2013). The rhetorics of health and medicine: Inventional possibilities for scholarship and engaged practice. *POROI: An Interdisciplinary Journal of Rhetorical Analysis and Invention, 9*(1), Article 17.

Segal, J. Z. (1994). Patient compliance, the rhetoric of rhetoric, and the theory of persuasion. *Rhetoric Society Quarterly, 23*(3–4), 90–102.

Segal, J. Z. (1997). Public discourse and public policy: Some ways that metaphor constrains health (care). *Journal of Medical Humanities, 18*(4), 217–231.

Segal, J. Z. (2005). *Heath and the rhetoric of medicine.* Carbondale: Southern Illinois University Press.

Segal, J. Z. (2007). "Compliance" to "concordance": A critical view. *Journal of Medical Humanities, 28*(2), 81–96.

Segal, J. Z. (2009). Rhetoric of health and medicine. In A. A. Lunsford (Ed.), *The Sage handbook of rhetorical studies* (pp. 227–245). Los Angeles, CA: Sage.

Seigel, M. (2014). *The rhetoric of pregnancy.* Chicago, IL: The University of Chicago Press.

Selber, S. (2010). A rhetoric of electronic instruction sets. *Technical Communication Quarterly, 19*(2), 95–117.

Selinger, E., & Mix, J. (2006). On interactional expertise: Pragmatic and ontological considerations. In E. Selinger & R. P. Crease (Eds.), *The philosophy of expertise* (pp. 302–321). New York, NY: Columbia University Press.

Selzer, J. (2004). Rhetorical analysis: Understanding how texts persuade readers. In C. Bazerman & P. Prior (Eds.), *What writing does and how it does it: An introduction to analyzing texts and textual practices* (pp. 279–307). Mahwah, NJ: Lawrence Erlbaum Associates.

Shakespeare, T. (1996). Disability, identity and difference. In C. Barnes & G. Mercer (Eds.), *Exploring the divide* (pp. 94–113). Leeds, UK: The Disability Press.

Shannon, C. E., & Weaver, W. (1948). A mathematical theory of communication. *The Bell System Technical Journal, 27,* 379–423.

Sklaroff, S. (2012 January 9). Diabetes affects millions; society should not stigmatize its victims. *The Washington Post.* Retrieved from: https://www.washingtonpost.com

Skyler, J. S., Bergenstal, R., Bonow, R. O., Buse, J., Deedwania, P., Gale, E. A. M., Sherwin, R. S. (2009). Intensive gylcemic control and the prevention of cardiovascular events: Implications of the ACCORD, ADVANCE, and VA Diabetes Trials. *Diabetes Care, 32*(1), 187–192.

Slack, J. D. (1989). Contextualizing technology. In B. Dervin, L. Grossberg, & E. A. Wartella (Eds.), *Rethinking communication: Paradigm exemplars* (pp. 329–345). Thousand Oaks, CA: Sage.

Slack, J. D. (2005). The theory and method of articulation in cultural studies. In D. Morley & K. Chen (Eds.), *Stuart Hall: Critical dialogues in cultural studies* (pp. 113–129). New York, NY: Routledge.

Slack, J. D., Miller, D. J., & Doak, J. (1993). The technical communicator as author: Meaning, power, authority. *Journal of Business and Technical Communication, 7*(1), 12–36.

Slattery, S. (2007). Undistributing work through writing: How technical writers manage texts in complex information environments. *Technical Communication Quarterly, 16*(3), 311–324.

Snider, B. (2006). The certainty of numbers. *Poetry Mountain.* Retrieved from: http://www.poetrymountain.com/authors/brucesnider.html

Soja, E. (1989). *Postmodern geographies: The reassertion of space in critical social theory.* London, UK: Verso.

Soja, E. W. (1996). *Thirdspace: Journeys to Los Angeles and other real-and-imagined places.* Oxford, UK: Blackwell Publishing.

Sontag, S. (1978). *Illness as metaphor.* New York, NY: Farrar, Straus, & Giroux.

Sorrell, K. (2014). The growing need for shared decision-making tools and how medical writers are equipped to meet it. *AMWA Journal, 29*(4), 148–150.

Sowards, S. (2010). Rhetorical agency as haciendo caras and differential consciousness through lens of gender, race, ethnicity, and class: An examination of Dolores Huerta's rhetoric. *Communication Theory, 20,* 223–247.

Spafford, M. M., Schryer, C. F., & Lingard, L. (2008). The rhetoric of patient voice: Reported talk with patients in referral and consultation letters. *Communication and Medicine, 5*(2), 93–104.

Spafford, M. M., Schryer, C. F., Mian, M., & Lingard, L. (2006). Look who's talking: Teaching and learning using the genre of medical case presentations. *Journal of Business and Technical Communication, 20*(2), 121–158.

Sparling, K. M. (2009, February 5). Vlogging while low. *Six Until Me.* Retrieved from http://sixuntilme.com/2009/02/vlogging_while_low.html

Sparling, K. M. (2011, November 14). My Dexcom sleeps nude. *Six Until Me.* Retrieved from http://sixuntilme.com/2011/11/my_dexcom_sleeps_nude.html

Spilka, R. (Ed.). (1993). *Writing in the workplace: New research perspectives.* Carbondale: Southern Illinois University Press.

Spinuzzi, C. (2003). *Tracing genres through organizations: A sociocultural approach to information design.* Cambridge, MA: MIT Press

Spinuzzi, C. (2007). Guest editor's introduction: Technical communication in the age of distributed work. *Technical Communication Quarterly, 16*(3), 265–277.

Spinuzzi, C. (2008). *Network: Theorizing knowledge work in telecommunication.* Cambridge, MA: Cambridge University Press.

Spinuzzi, C. (2012). Working alone together: Coworking as emergent collaborative activity. *Journal of Business and Technical Communication, 26*(4), 399–441.

Spinuzzi, C., Hart-Davidson, W., & Zachry, M. (2006). Chains and ecologies: Methodological notes toward a communicative-mediational model of technologically mediated writing. In *Proceedings of the 24th Annual ACM International Conference on Design of Communication* (pp. 43–50). Myrtle Beach, SC: Association for Computing Machinery.

Spivak, G. C. (1993). *Outside in the teaching machine.* New York, NY: Routledge.

The StayWell Company (2015). *Living well with diabetes: A self-care workbook.* Retrieved from: http://ada-ksw.com/diabetes/#/1/

Stimson, G. V. (1974). Obeying doctor's orders: A view from the other side. *Social Science & Medicine, 8*(2), 97–104.

Stone, D. B. (1961). A study of the incidences and causes of poor control in patients with diabetes mellitus. *The American Journal of Medical Sciences, 241*(4), 436–442.

Stone, M. S. (1997). In search of patient agency in the rhetoric of diabetes care. *Technical Communication Quarterly, 6*(2), 201–217.

Stormer, N. (2004). Articulation: A working paper on rhetoric and taxis. *Quarterly Journal of Speech, 90*(3), 257–284.

Sverrisson, A. (2001). Translation networks, knowledge brokers and novelty construction: Pragmatic environmentalism in Sweden. *Acta Sociologica, 44,* 313–327.

Swarts, J., & Kim, L. (2009). Guest editors' introduction: New technological spaces. *Technical Communication Quarterly, 18*(3), 211–223.

Tannen, D. (1989). *Talking voices: Repetition, dialogue, and imagery in conversational discourse.* Cambridge, MA: Harvard University Press.

Terrill, R. (2011). Mimesis, duality, and rhetorical education. *Rhetoric Society Quarterly, 41*(4), 295–315.

Thompson, G., & Ye, Y. (1991). Evaluation in the verbs used in academic papers. *Applied Linguistics, 12,* 365–382.

Timmermans, S., & Berg, M. (2003). *The gold standard: The challenge of evidence-based medicine and standardization in healthcare.* Philadelphia, PA: Temple University Press.

Trostle, J. A. (1988). Medical compliance as ideology. *Social Science & Medicine, 27,* 1299–1308.

TuDiabetes. (2016). Our editorial policy. *TuDiabetes.org.* Retrieved from http://www.tudiabetes.org/our-editorial-policy/

Turner, V. (1967). *The forest of symbols: Aspects of Ndembu ritual.* Ithaca, NY: Cornell University Press.

Turner, V. (1974). *Dramas, fields, and metaphors: Symbolic action in human society.* Ithaca, NY: Cornell University Press.

UK Prospective Diabetes Study (UKPDS) Group. (1998). Intensive blood-glucose control with sulphonylureas or insulin compared with conventional treatment and risk of complications in patients with type 2 diabetes. *Lancet, 352,* 837–853.

U.S. Department of Veteran Affairs. (2013). A1C test. *va.gov.* Retrieved from http://www.mirecc.va.gov/cih-visn2/Documents/Patient_Education_Handouts/A1C_Test_Version_3.pdf

Van Gennep, A., (1960). *The rites of passage.* Chicago, IL: The University of Chicago Press.

Vatz, R. E. (1973). The myth of the rhetorical situation. *Philosophy and Rhetoric, 6*(3), 154–161.

Vatz, R. E. (1981). Vatz on Patton and Bitzer. *Quarterly Journal of Speech, 67*(1), 95–99.

Vatz, R. E. (2006). Rhetoric and psychiatry: A Szaszian perspective on a political case study. *Current Psychology, 25*(3), 173–181.

Vatz, R. E. (2009). The mythical status of situational rhetoric: Implications for rhetorical critics' relevance in the public arena. *The Review of Communication, 9*(1), 1–5.

Vivian, B. (2000). The threshold of the self. *Philosophy and Rhetoric, 3*(4), 303–318.

Vološinov, V. N. (1973). *Marxism and the philosophy of language* (L. Matejka & I. R. Titunik, Trans.). London, UK: Seminar Press.

Walkowski, D. (1991). Working successfully with technical experts—from their perspective. *Technical Communication, 38,* 65–67.

Warf, B. (2009). From surfaces to networks. In B. Warf & S. Arias (Eds.), *The spatial turn: Interdisciplinary perspectives* (pp. 59–76). New York, NY: Routledge.

Warf, B., & Arias, S. (Eds.). (2009). *The spatial turn: Interdisciplinary perspectives.* New York, NY: Routledge.

Warne, C. (2006). *Aristotle's Nicomachean Ethics: Reader's guide.* London, UK: Continuum International Publishing Group.

Warner, M. (2002). Publics and counterpublics. *Public Culture, 14*(1), 49–71.

Weaver, R. (1953). *The ethics of rhetoric.* Davis, CA: Hermagoras.

Weaver, R. (2001). Language is sermonic. In P. Bizzell & B. Herzberg (Eds.), *The rhetorical tradition: Readings from classical times to the present* (pp. 1351–1360). Boston, MA: Bedford/St Martin's.

Weinberger, D. (2012). *Too big to know: Rethinking knowledge now that the facts aren't the facts, experts are everywhere, and the smartest person in the room is the room.* New York, NY: Basic Books.

Wenger, E. (2006). Communities of practice: A brief introduction. Retrieved from http://wenger-trayner.com/introduction-to-communities-of-practice/

Winsor, D. A. (1999). Genre and activity systems: The role of documentation in maintaining and changing engineering activity systems. *Written Communication, 16*(2), 200–224.

Winsor, D. A. (2000). Ordering work—Blue-collar literacy and the political nature of genre. *Written Communication, 17*(2), 155–184.

Winsor, D. A. (2001). Learning to do knowledge work in systems of distributed cognition. *Journal of Business and Technical Communication, 15*(1), 5–28.

Winsor, D. A. (2003). *Writing power: Communication in an engineering center.* Albany: State University of New York Press.

Winsor, D. (2006). Using writing to structure agency: An examination of engineers' practice. *Technical Communication Quarterly, 15*(4), 411–430.

Wolf, D. L. (Ed.). (1996). *Situating feminist dilemmas in fieldwork.* Oxford, UK: Westview Press.

World Health Organization (WHO). (1980). *Report of the expert committee on diabetes* (Technical Report Series No. 646). Geneva, Switzerland: World Health Organization.

Yancey, K. B. (2011). Writing agency, writing practices, writing pasts and futures. *College Composition and Communication, 62*(3), 415–419.

Zarefsky, D., Miller-Tutzauer, C., & Tutzauer, F. E. (1984). Reagan's safety net for the truly needy: The rhetorical uses of definition. *Central States Speech Journal, 35,* 113–119.

INDEX

A1C, 3, 3n6, 27–28, 27n3, 33, 37, 64–65, 69, 113, 162

ADA (American Diabetes Association), 2–4, 23–27, 34, 41, 47, 57, 59, 76–77, 81–83, 85, 111, 143, 162–63

ADA, *Standards of Medical Care,* 2n3, 3n7, 22, 35, 82, 86–87, 130–31, 137, 143, 146

adherence, 16, 122

Affordable Care Act, 158

agency, 2–13, 15–19, 21–24, 26, 28–31, 45–47, 51, 66–68, 71–72, 74–75, 99–100, 123–25, 148–55, 158–59; as authorship, 8; collapse of, 11; dis-articulating, 30; locating, 61, 149; need to redefine, 16; as possession, 8; re-articulating, 17, 50, 149, 151, 153 155, 157, 159, 161, 163, 165; as relational, 8, 26, 118; and structure, 151; temporary, 125; user, 9. *See also* patient agency; rhetorical agency

AHRQ (Agency for Health-Care Research and Quality), 55, 166

ambiguity, 61, 111, 136

articulations, 11–13, 16, 19, 21, 24, 45–46, 50, 59, 61, 74, 117, 120, 123–24, 149–51; agential, 125; multiple, 13, 117; practice of, 11–12, 12n26, 100; simultaneous, 136; temporary, 50, 66, 123

articulation theory, 12

artificial pancreas, 45

assemblage, 11

audience, intended, 158

authority, 17, 29, 45, 62, 70, 93, 106–7, 114, 128–29, 140, 145, 186; authorial, 58; med-ical, 31, 53, 55, 72, 85, 127, 153; medical online, 146; narrative, 114; resistance to, 9, 9n24; scientific, 147

authorship, 8, 71n15, 114, 114n8, 117, 117n12

autonomy, 2, 11, 18, 31, 92, 123, 150, 181; and freedom, 17

bad diabetic, 66. *See also under* patients

balance, 42, 64, 162–64; and diet, 162–63

Banting, Frederick, 44

BCG (bacille Calmette-Guerin) vaccine, 97

betweenity, 61–62, 74

blame, 16, 31, 37, 39, 67, 68, 94; discourse of, 66

blameworthy, 67

blood glucose. *See* blood sugar

blood glucose level. *See* blood sugar levels

blood glucose meter, 6, 9, 13, 15, 31, 33, 35, 39, 45–46, 56–58, 74, 76, 87, 99, 112, 162, 167

blood glucose monitoring, 56, 35, 48, 167, 169; remote, 98

blood glucose numbers, nondiabetic, 164

blood sugar, 3–4, 15, 18, 32–37, 42, 57, 74–79, 84–85, 87–89, 95, 102–3, 112–13, 128–29, 132, 135–36, 164, 167–69; fasting, 27; fluctuations, 167; goal, 162; monitor, 19, 53, 56–57, 68, 98; symptoms of low, 59, 89–90; test, 3, 35, 53, 58, 81, 91, 162, 169

blood sugar numbers, 1, 5, 9, 18–19, 22, 28, 32–34, 37, 42, 53, 56–57, 59, 66, 74, 77, 79, 88–89, 91, 95, 162, 167–68; high, 14, 34, 44, 57, 64, 78, 90, 99, 103, 168–69; low,